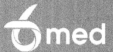 

UCAT CRASH COURSE

CW00410138

In A Nutshell

We know you're busy. So here's the essential information about the 6med BMAT Crash Course.

1. It's a one-day course, which runs from 10am – 5:30pm most weekends from June – September each year.

2. The course was created by Oxbridge medics and is led by an instructor who is a medical student at one of the top universities in the country. The course is priced at £129 per student.

3. Each student gets a copy of our 300-page A4 course book.

Course Overview

People often describe UCAT as an exam that "cannot be prepared for". We disagree. It's true that the style of the test means that there aren't any facts to learn (unlike BMAT), but you can absolutely familiarize yourself with the different sections, and practice techniques that will get you through each question in a timely fashion. These techniques are what we'll be teaching you on the UCAT Crash Course.

We spend around 1.5 hours on each of the 4 main UCAT sections (Verbal Reasoning, Quantitative Reasoning, Abstract Reasoning and Situational Judgment). We spend 30 minutes going over strategy and technique, and an hour on doing timed practice questions in an interactive fashion. See course details & timetable.

Our experienced instructors (all current medical students) make sure that everyone's clear on how to tackle the questions using the best strategies.

Course Reviews

Hundreds and hundreds of students have attended our courses and loved them.

I would just like to say a huge huge thank you for helping me obtain all 4 medicine offers! I attended your UCAT and Interview courses (which would not have been possible without your generous bursaries!), along with having my personal statement checked. All 3 100% enabled me to obtain interviews and then offers. Everyone who I met was super friendly and up for banter aha which made the whole process a little less daunting!".

Haya (Medicine Applicant)

Course Handbook

www.6med.co.uk

www.exams.ninja

Published by *6med*
www.6med.co.uk

About the Author

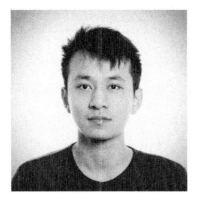

James is a junior doctor and one of the founders of 6med. He studied neuroscience at UCL alongside creating a number of our UCAT resources - including this book!

About the Editor

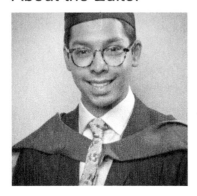

Inayat is a fourth year medical student in London. He initially did a Science degree, achieving a first with honours before joining a graduate MBBS course. Having started tutoring whilst in sixth form he has a keen interest in education and now leads courses for 6med.

When he's not on the wards or in the library, Inayat can be found trying out new coffee shops, running or listening to a podcast.

Collaborators

We're a close-knit team of medical students, junior doctors, future dentists, and late night takeaway enthusiasts here at 6med! So we wanted to thank everyone who helped put this book together with hints, tips, and generously donating their time and question-writing imagination for you to use!

Christopher Dorman
University College, London
LLB (Hons)

Aqib Chaudry
Imperial College, London
MBBS, BSc (Hons)

Haroon Ahmed
Queen's College, Cambridge
MBBS, BSc (Hons)

Ali Abdaal
Emmanuel College, Cambridge
MBBS, BSc (Hons)

If you'd like to get in touch - just check the contact page on the website for our most up-to-date information.

We put a lot of time into writing this, and would also really appreciate it if you didn't photocopy it and give it to your mates :)

This is a placeholder page. It will be replaced with a beautiful full colour ad for UCAT Ninja that Adi has created.

You might think we could take this page out of the manuscript entirely, but no.

If we do that, the book has one fewer pages than it is supposed to it, which screws up the page numbering.

And the contents page

And make Amazon Kindle Direct Publishing angry.

So instead, after the manuscript has been converted to pdf.

We extract this page using a pdf compiler

And insert the new page.

So please don't screw around with this page!

Contents

Introduction

About Us

Hello, and welcome to UCAT Crash Course! We know this is an important time, and are delighted that you've allowed us to be a part of your journey.

The medical admissions process is fun, but it isn't easy - our aim is to make this particular step (the UCAT) as painless as it can be, and to maximize your score in it. As a team of medical students, we've all been through the process and come out alive - we want to impart our skills, knowledge and experience to help you do the same. Best of luck!

Who are we?

We're a team of medical students from some of the UK's top universities. Our team is made up of graphic designers, web developers, Taekwondo instructors, concert pianists, close-up magicians, stage singers, and so much more. Our friendship and love of teaching has allowed us to work together to form this company (6med) while juggling our university academic and social lives, and it's been an amazing ride for all of us.

6med started in 2013 with the BMAT Crash Course. It was supposed to be a fun little job to teach 2-3 courses in the summer holidays and make a bit of money on the side. Over the years, it's grown bigger than we could have ever imagined, to the point where we're teaching over a thousand students each year, with many more thousands accessing our materials online and buying this textbook!

While our company has grown and our student numbers (and satisfaction ratings) steadily increased, our mission has stayed the same - to provide the most effective, yet most affordable, preparation in the world.

Why do we do what we do?

We like the fact that medical school admission is such a competitive process, but don't like the edge that having lots of money gives you over the competition. At 6med, we aim to "level the playing field", so to speak. Our courses cost a fraction of the price of others, and we provide a huge number of bursaries for students unable to afford them. We think that medical school admission should be based on ability, potential and motivation - not how much money your parents have.

How do we do it?

So now that you know a bit about us, you might be wondering how we do it. There's no easy answer to that - it's just a case of spending hundreds of hours creating the website, creating the course, writing this textbook, marketing, etc. Once all that's been sorted, all that's left to do is to teach the actual courses, which is quite straightforward compared to all the work that goes into the setup.

We hope you gain something from this book, and please, if you can think of any ways in which we can improve, tell us in person, or email us (anonymously or otherwise) after you've finished. This book is designed for you, and we'll do everything we can to make sure that it's the best it can possibly be.

Aims

The UCAT isn't content based, so we won't be barraging you with theory. Importantly, we want you to take a serious look at how you're approaching the UCAT and break down the process step by step - many students go into the exam with bad habits, tackling questions slowly and inefficiently. There is a clear approach (which we'll give you) that will increase your chances of achieving a strong score - but it's up to you to you to take advantage of the methods and to practice effectively.

We're going to spend the majority of the time covering the five assessed subtests (VR, QR, AR, SJT, DM). Within each section, we'll go over the most important things that you can apply straight away to your practice and hopefully use to boost your score on the day of the exam. For each chapter, we'll run through the basic 'strategy' first - this consists of useful tips and advice you should use in your practice. After this, your tutors will guide you through the 'workbook': this is an interactive course after all, so you'll be expected to do the questions under exam conditions and contribute to the class discussion. Ask your tutors anything you want - they'll be running through the best approach for each question, and also adding any extra advice they may have.

Here are just a few of the most important things we'll deal with:

Basic information and Format
This is an important area - we'll be going over the basic format for each section and make sure you understand what's being tested. There have been a few new changes to the specification over the last few years, so it's important you know exactly what's going to come up on test-day.

Timing and Pacing
Without a doubt, the strict time limit is one of the biggest challenges candidates face. Many test-takers find themselves losing time on each set as the test goes on, and by the end, they may not finish and miss out on easy marks. Most candidates won't have a problem solving the majority of questions, but the main problems are a result of the intense pressure and lack of time. This course will lay down the best timings you should stick to for each section, and we'll try to advise you on the best ways to optimize your time on questions.

Question Categories
Having an awareness of the different question categories allows you to anticipate the commonly tested areas, and also helps you focus on your weaknesses during your practice. The more you practice with the different categories, the more familiar you'll be with the exam, and the faster you'll answer each question.

Preparation and Practice

Having a strong approach and strategy is one thing, but putting it into practice requires a bit of extra thought. Your tutors, and this book, will give you some ideas to get started, but you have to be smart with your practice if you want to make the most out of the strategies. Look through our preparation, strategy and practice chapters, and try to be as effective as possible during your study sessions. Remember, the hard work you put in now will pay off in the long run.

How to Use This Book

Obviously, which bits of the book you focus on will depend on what it is about the personal statement you find the most tricky. There are some general tips though:

Be prepared to change your approach.

Many test-takers go about doing questions their 'own way' - even though they've never handled a psychometric test before. Although there are several ways to approach the UCAT, the best methods will help you optimize the way you spend your time on each question. Some students feel uncomfortable changing the way they tackle questions - try to stick to the strategies we teach you and take a look at our worked solutions. If you feel uncomfortable or confused, let your tutor know!

Apply the strategies to your practice.

You may feel overloaded with information, at least initially, but after a week or so, you'll feel more comfortable using the methods on this course and will inevitably see results. There are a number of things that you can use straight away - for example, time-saving techniques for QR, speed reading for VR, and using the SSSPN approach for AR. Other things may take a bit longer, but how well you integrate the strategies will depend on the quality and quantity of your practice (which we'll help you on).

Keep this book handy.

You may need to refer back to various bits in the book or any annotations you've made - the methods in this course should form a solid foundation for future practice, so you should use it throughout your study.

Top Tips from the Team

As a kind of introduction, we wanted to include our personal top tips.

Sam Darrington, 6med Course Lead

Hi!

Preparing to sit the UCAT can be a really daunting experience, and to help with that we've packed this book full of strategies, ideas, information, and guidance on how to do as well as possible. All of it is relevant, so it's well worth reading through, but for me and my brigade of UCAT veterans, there are four key points that we'd be keen to stress:

1. Practice, practice, practice.

   The **most** important thing you can do is practice UCAT questions. This book is full of things you can practice and try out, run through all of them. Ultimately, the book has a limited number of questions (because we can only print so many before it starts getting too heavy to carry around everywhere, which you all do, right?) When you have run through the questions in the book, and the UCAT website, ukcat.ninja has *thousands* of practice questions, and realistic past papers.

2. Take your exam before school starts.

   You have a lot of leeway, usually, in when you take the UCAT. Lots of people end up rushing in October when they're also busy with school and BMAT and it's an unnecessary challenge. Take it in the summer holidays, and you can enjoy your summer and be able to focus entirely on schoolwork when you're back.

3. Set aside clear time to study.

   If you are practicing regularly, and using this guide, the UCAT does not need more than a few hours of practice a day to ace. At least three weeks before your exam set aside a specific time each day dedicated to studying (if you do this in the summer holidays this should be even easier!)

4. Pay attention to your weaknesses.

   Your brain needs exercise like the rest of you, in each study session, make a note of what you are finding the trickiest and work on strengthening your thinking in that area.

Working with these in mind will go a long way to helping you quickly falling into a work schedule that maximises your UCAT skills.

1. Time management.

This is so important, try and pay attention to how much time you spend (practicing for the exam, like Sam said) in the exam. You have time limits for each section which you must stick to.

2. Learn to drop questions you can't do.

You've got to work through the exam really quickly. If you prepare with this guide, chances are there won't be a lot of questions you can't do, but if you find one *skip it.* If you get to the end with time to spare, go back and check, but otherwise, try to avoid wasting time on a question you don't know how to answer once you've finished reading it.

3. Learn how to quickly answer questions.

The follow on from the above point is that you should learn to carry out mental maths very quickly. You want to be able to tear through the Quantitative Reasoning section.

4. Read the news.

Try to stick to more reputable news sources, as well as topical magazines like New Scientist. This has two advantages; you have more knowledge about current affairs (which helps at interview) and you can use these to practice quickly summarising articles as Verbal Reasoning practice.

5. Don't panic.

Try to get loads of rest before the big day, eat a big breakfast, drink lots of water, and in the exam try your best to stay calm.

"Don't be nervous" is the worst advice in the world, and I remember how stressful the exam is, but panicking really, really doesn't help!

General Information

You probably already know a lot of this! But it can be useful to have it all in one place!

So, what is the UCAT?

Over the past few years, more and more highly qualified students are applying to medical school. As a result, the University Clinical Aptitude Test is used by many medical schools to give a better indication of the applicants that are more likely to become good clinicians.

The UCAT is a 2 hour psychometric test - a test that attempts to objectively measure aspects of your mental ability or personality. Psychometric tests are used not only for medical/dental entry, but by employers in a diverse range of industries; it allows for a direct comparison between different candidates.

The UCAT tests a wide range of skills, reflected in the five main subtests:
1. Verbal reasoning
2. Decision making
3. Quantitative reasoning
4. Abstract reasoning
5. Situational Judgement Test

Keep in mind, unlike the BMAT and the exams you've done at school, you don't need much prior knowledge - this isn't a content-based exam. Instead, the UCAT requires the test-taker to have robust numerical skills, an ability to evaluate and scrutinize written information, skills in pattern identification, and a capability to make decisions in situations of uncertainty. In effect, the primary aim of the UCAT is to measure underlying ability, and not the differing quality of education applicants receive. At the same time, don't be swayed by thinking this is an IQ test you can't prepare for - you can prepare for the UCAT, but you'll need to prepare differently: a stronger emphasis should be placed on practice and strategy, not revision.

Summary

- The UCAT is a psychometric test measuring five main areas: Verbal reasoning, Decision making, Quantitative reasoning, Abstract reasoning and Situational Judgement Test
- The UCAT is not a content-based exam - it measures underlying ability, but you can prepare for it and maximise your score.

How is the UCAT scored?

The UCAT isn't negatively marked, so take advantage of this by never leaving a question blank. The number of raw correct responses are scaled, from a minimum score of 300 to a maximum score of 900. The total score can therefore range from 900 to 3600.

The translation from your raw mark to your UCAT score is a complicated process. When doing mock exams or practice questions, you can never know what score you'll get just by looking at the number of correct responses you've made. Putting it simply, raw scores are scaled and translated from 300 to 900 based on the number of correct responses given by a designated group of 'test-takers'. A score of 600 corresponds to the mean raw mark in this test-taker pool, and one standard deviation either side corresponds to scores of 500 and 700. As a result, the raw mark you get on test-day will be 'adjusted' (in comparison to this group of test-takers) to give your final UCAT score.

Here are some statistics (from 2017). It's important to remember that you don't need to get every single question correct to achieve a score of 900. In practice, you can get a few questions wrong and still achieve a very high score. This means you shouldn't slow yourself down on the harder questions and have a mindset of quickly discarding and deciding in order to maximize easier marks elsewhere.

Average overall score	2,540
Verbal Reasoning	570
Quantitative Reasoning	695
Abstract Reasoning	629
Decision Making	647
Average section score	635
Excellent score	Above 700
Outstanding score (>80% correct)	Above 800
Exceptional score	900

How is the UCAT used?

Different universities use your UCAT score in different ways. Some place a larger emphasis on the UCAT - for example, Sheffield recommends a minimum UCAT threshold score of 2600 (650 average). Other medical schools use the UCAT as part of a wider application and will take everything into account.

Medical schools may use your UCAT score in three key ways:

- When they need to make a tough decision between two similar candidates.
- As part of wider application (given a percentage weighting).
- To compare against a threshold score for entry.

The five subtests

It's a good idea to keep an overview of the test in mind while working through questions or it's easy to get too involved in one question and before you know it you're running out of time for that section.

Section	Timing	Format
VR	*Total:* 22 minutes Breakdown: 1 minute (instructions), 21 minutes (questions)	Total questions: 44Q *Breakdown:* 11 passages (4Qs each) Types: 'SBA' sets (4 statements), 'True-false' sets
DM	*Total:* 32 minutes Breakdown: 1 minute (instructions), 31 minutes (questions)	Total questions: 29Q
QR	*Total:* 26 minutes Breakdown: 1 minute (instructions), 25 minutes (questions)	Total questions: 36Q *Breakdown:* 9 sets (4Q each)
AR	*Total:* 13 minutes Breakdown: 1 minute (instructions), 12 minutes (questions)	Total Questions: 50Q *Breakdown:* 10 sets (5Q each) Types: Type 1 (Set A/B/Neither) Type 2 (Test shape that follows sequence) Type 3 (missing test shape in statement) Type 4 (test shape matching either Set A or B)
SJT	*Total:* 27 minutes Breakdown: 1 minute (instructions), 26 minutes (questions)	Total questions: 66Q *Breakdown:* 22 scenarios (2-3Qs each)

What exactly is each section testing?

Verbal Reasoning

This section will require you to read through a passage of information and then answer a series of four questions about what you have read. Essentially, this is a comprehension test. You will need to scrutinise and evaluate written information, both in the passage and in the questions themselves. The length of the passages and the strict time limit means that students often feel a great deal of pressure on this subtest.

Decision Making

You will be tested on your ability to reach a decision or conclusion through the application of logic, and to evaluate arguments and analyse statistics

Quantitative Reasoning

The primary goal of this section is to test problem-solving ability. You are expected to know mathematical concepts to a GCSE level, although only a select few areas are examined (the exam will not cover the entire mathematics GCSE syllabus). Once again, the strict time limits make this section difficult.

Abstract Reasoning

This section requires you to detect a pattern or sequence from a series of boxes which contain shapes. The questions asked are somewhat similar to those in an IQ test; if you have not taken one of these, there is a fair chance that you won't have seen this type of question before. Taking the correct approach can make this section a great deal less complicated than it may otherwise seem.

Situational Judgment

In this section, a short scenario is given in which there is some kind of moral dilemma. You must assess how appropriate certain courses of action are in response to this, or how important certain considerations will be when determining a response.

Useful information

Signing up & Booking

- Sign up and book the UCAT at www.ucat.ac.uk. You'll need to complete a short questionnaire containing questions regarding you and your parents. Don't worry, this information is confidential and kept safely by the UCAT consortium.
- Before booking the test, ensure you have an idea of which universities require the UCAT and how they use it.
- The help control demand, the fee is generally lower for both UK and EU students in the Summer than in September. It's for you to find the right balance between preparation time and cost saving.
- The fee for tests taken outside the EU is generally higher.

Bursary

- Check if you're eligible for a bursary (see www.ucat.ac.uk/registration/bursaries/) - and make sure that you apply before the deadline with any supporting information.
- You will receive a voucher code if your application is successful, and you can use it even if you need to reschedule.

Special Arrangements

- Check if you're unsure if your eligible for special arrangements in the exam (UCAT Special Educational Needs) (see www.ucat.ac.uk/registration/candidates-with-disabilities/).
- The UCATSEN will give you additional time, and eligible candidates may have dyslexia, ADHD or working memory deficit, among other disabilities and conditions. Contact the UCAT Consortium if you're unsure you're eligible.
- If you require specific test-centre arrangements (for a disability or medical condition), contact the UCAT consortium directly.

Exempt Students

- If you're planning on taking the UCAT outside the UK, check the country has a test centre, and if not, you may be exempt from taking the UCAT.
- If you believe you may be exempt from taking the UCAT for any other reason (medical grounds, etc.) - contact the UCAT consortium directly.

Preparation

What Preparation is Required?

For many of you, the UCAT is an intimidating part of the application procedure, but by the end of the day, you'll have the necessary skills to overcome this hurdle. While the exam techniques and methods of revision you needed for GCSEs and A-levels have been built up over the years, the UCAT is a new challenge many of you haven't come across before - this is why effective, targeted preparation is so important. You must approach the UCAT from a different angle and plan appropriately in order to have the best chance of success.

Although the UCAT is an aptitude test, with good preparation and focused practice, you'll get a strong score. We've seen countless students score below average in their first sitting, and after better preparation and more practice, score in the high 700s the next year. If you put in the hard graft today, you'll save yourself a lot of time and hopefully secure the offer you want. So how do I prepare for the UCAT, and what exactly am I working on?

To put it in a nutshell, success in any psychometric test can be distilled into the following:

1. **Focus on the data types**

   This is all about anticipation. Before you walk into any exam room, you should know the type of questions that will come up. However, we mean much more than simply having a rough idea of the different questions: you should be comfortable with every question category in all five subtests, and have a clear approach for almost every question that can be tested. For example, in QR there are several question categories that are commonly tested (geometry, percentage change, etc.) - knowing what comes up (and what doesn't) will save you time and help you target your practice.

2. **Find ways of saving time**

   Timing can make or break test-takers. We've seen intelligent students score consistently below 600 because they utilize inefficient methods and are simply too slow. Saving time can mean having an efficient strategy, finding quicker ways of solving questions (mental maths, speed reading, etc.) or strategically skipping questions. Throughout the course, we'll be drilling into your head the most important ways to save time.

3. **Automate your test-taking**

   The UCAT, unlike your school exams, isn't a content-based exam. In essence, you're developing skills and learning to apply effective strategies in each subtest. Preparation comes before automation, and this course will give you the tools you need to start. With enough practice, you'll be able to anticipate various test challenges, swiftly locate relevant data, and know exactly which techniques to apply. It doesn't take as long as you think to achieve automation, research suggests it's possible after just a few days of intense practice.

4. **Increase your confidence**

   It's suggested performance is directly linked with a test-taker's level of confidence. A student who expects to succeed is more likely to succeed than a student who does not. One of the biggest obstacles to UCAT success is a lack of confidence, but the best way to increase your confidence in anything is by getting good at it. Don't cram your UCAT practice, take your time, and consistently work at it. If you've put the work in, and have applied the strategies outlined in our course, you should be confident on the day of your exam.

How accurately does the UCAT reflect my ability?

The UCAT doesn't test you on curricular content (unlike the BMAT), and so experts construct questions that aim to test 'cognitive ability'. In theory, measures of natural ability shouldn't be affected by the amount of practice or preparation put in - but from our experience, this has proven not to be the case for the UCAT.

We believe that the UCAT, to an extent, is correlated with an individual's natural ability, but without smart preparation and practice, the test-taker will not achieve his or her highest possible score. If you want to do the best you possibly can, make sure you take the time to plan out your preparation and practice using the best strategies. Of course, some individuals do attain very high scores without much practice or preparation, but who's to say they couldn't have achieved an even higher score with effective preparation.

Whatever your ability, it doesn't change the way you prepare for the UCAT - focus on your weaknesses and what you can change and stop worrying if you're good enough.

Your Study Plan

A lot of students don't have a plan for the UCAT - and that's something you must not do. You must have a plan for your preparation. Cramming may work for some exams at school, but the UCAT requires consistent practice. Don't be fooled by people who put in minimal work and achieve high scores. Just because the UCAT is unfamiliar, don't take it any less seriously than any other exam. Remember, hope for the best and prepare for the worst. As soon as you know you're going to take the UCAT, the first thing you should do is draw up a plan.

An effective study plan is much more than a timetable. It defines an approach that cultivates productive learning and effective practice, as well as dealing with any problems that may arise during the study period.

1. **Decide how much time you're willing to dedicate to UCAT practice.**

   This depends on how early you start. If you have 2 months ahead of you, nobody is expecting you to work every day. However, a month before test-day, we do recommend you put in daily practice if you can - at least one or two hours. The amount of work you put in really depends on you, but whatever you do, make sure you avoid excuses and stick to your plan.

   Remember, focus is everything. If you're unfocused, you may make silly mistakes and fail to mimic real exam conditions. Don't overdo your sessions, and keep them as productive as possible. At the same time, it's important to remember the exam is 2 hours long and that you need to be focused throughout. Closer to the day of the exam, aim to replicate these conditions by doing full-length mock exams under strict timing.

2. **Don't trust your memory - write it down.**

   Some students can get distracted quite easily, and unless you write down your plan, you'll probably forget to fit in UCAT practice consistently. If this means setting a reminder on your phone to revise at a set time each day, then so be it. Do whatever it takes to optimize your score.

   We recommend you keep a 'practice journal'. As mundane as it may sound, the key to getting into the right frame of mind, or achieve 'flow', is to have clear intentions, i.e. knowing what to do and when to do it.

   You can write down something as simple as:

   Do UCAT study after dinner for 2 hours on Monday, Wednesday and Friday.

3. Plan ahead.

Keep a to-do list for your practice sessions so you know what you're working on, for example:

Monday - QR and VR
Wednesday - AR and DM
Friday - Mock Exam.

4. **Gather all your study materials.**

You're going to be using different resources, so keep everything in one place, and make sure you keep track of what you want to get through and by when.

Your UCAT practice should be consistent. The amount you do in one day isn't as important as how often you do it. You're essentially developing a new skill, so by doing a bit everyday (or every few days at the very least) you'll pick it up quicker: this is why planning ahead is important.

Productivity Tips

Being productive means making the most of your time. Unproductive UCAT study sessions may slow down your progress, and as a result, it may take you longer to internalize and automate strategies. If you're like most students, you may struggle with this area. The first step to becoming more productive is being honest with yourself - know when you're wasting your time, and take the appropriate action to ensure you're getting the most out of your study sessions.

Here are some research-based tips that may help you work more productively:

1. **Location, Location, Location**

Decide where you want to study. In your home? At the library? It doesn't matter as long as you know you won't get distracted. Once you've decided - try to stick with it, and keep all your UCAT resources there. Studies have shown that your hippocampus (in your brain) associates different types of focused work with particular places: if you're working on different things (or not working), consider dedicating a desk or table or section in your house for each.

2. **Create the habit**

It may be easier to get into a 'habit' of UCAT study, rather than forcing yourself every time you need to do it. Keep to the same routine: after dinner, before breakfast, after the gym, etc. Once a habit is formed, various elements from the environment can act as a cue to activate the behaviour, even without you having to make the decision.

Research suggests the best time to study is early in the morning and before you sleep. In the morning, you'll be fresh (hopefully) and have a clear mind. But in the end, you should know when you're at your best - protect those peak hours for your UCAT practice.

3. **Remove distractions**

Turn off your all your notifications. When you're working, your computer, phone or whatever gadgetry you have shouldn't be chiming every time you get a new message. We live in a world where everything is competing for our attention - but to be productive during our study time, we need to stop being in a mode where we're reacting to things. Don't get us wrong, these things are great in moderation, but they will seriously decrease the quality of your practice if you're constantly being distracted. A single notification can take your mind away from your work even if you don't choose to check it. As Time Ferris (productivity guru) puts it: 'Focus is a function, first and foremost, of limiting the number of options you give yourself for procrastinating'. Interestingly, in a study, high-school students whose classroom was situated closer to a noisy railroad line were a full academic year behind students with a quieter classroom.

4. **Set clear goals beforehand**

You should try to start your UCAT sessions knowing exactly what you need to work on or going to do - spend time in the previous session or night before defining your most important UCAT to- dos for the upcoming session. Writing things down also relieves any anxiety you might have and gives you something concrete to achieve. The more specific you are with your goals the better: it means you'll be more committed to doing it and forces you to actively reflect on your progress.

Strategy

Overview

In this chapter, we'll go over some of the more general, yet important, principles that underlies many of the techniques and methods taught later in the course. We can't emphasise enough the importance of time-management when thinking strategy. For every method of going about a question, when practicing, think if there is any way you can adjust your approach to minimise the time spent on each question. We will cover lots of these techniques in the upcoming chapters.

Marks and Timing

The UCAT isn't inherently a 'hard' test. To put it simply, the biggest challenge is getting as many questions right in the little time given to you. At the same time, don't sacrifice the accuracy of your answers for speed. On test-day, the best way to maximise the proportion of questions you get right is by knowing which questions to prioritize, when to prioritize, and when to skip.

Checking the timer and speed

Keeping an eye on the timer is important because it'll help you adjust your speed. Don't check the timer too much though - you can easily lose your train of thought halfway through a question if you're constantly looking up. Maintain a balance!

Halfway markers

Some test-takers who check the timer after every question may panic and rush through questions. It doesn't help to glance at the timer every 5 seconds, even though it's important to keep to a strict timing. With enough practice, you should know roughly when you have to move on. It may be a good idea to consider checking the timer at set points - the halfway marker (which you can find in our table) is a good place to quickly judge how you're managing your time, and if you need to speed up.

We've included some recommended timings over the page - it might seem impossible at first, but with practice you'll get there! And, if you follow our recommended timings, you'll actually have some spare time at the end (there'll be more on this later!)

Here is an overview of our recommended timings for each section:

Verbal Reasoning	
44 Questions	21 minutes
Passage (4 questions)	SBA: 2 minutes T/F: 1.5 minutes
Beginning of 6 Set (Halfway Marker)	11 minutes remaining
Quantitative Reasoning	
36 Questions	25 minutes
Set (4 questions)	2 minutes & 55 seconds
Beginning of 5 Set (HM)	13 minutes remaining (rounded up)
Abstract Reasoning	
50 Questions	12 min
Set (5 questions)	1 minute & 12 seconds
Beginning of 6 Set (HM)	6 minutes remaining
Situational Judgement	
66 Questions	26 minutes
1 question	23 seconds
By question 33 (HM)	13 minutes remaining
Decision Making	
29 questions	31 minutes
1 question	1 minute
By question 15	15 minutes remaining

Flag, Guess and Skip

In the UCAT, there's no negative marking, and you'll also come across a range of easier to more difficult questions. Each question is worth one mark - if you're stuck, don't spend too much time on the questions that you know will take too long. Instead, try discarding what you can, and then flag, guess and skip. Don't be afraid to make blind guesses and skip harder questions - very few students can accurately complete all questions in the UCAT. The best students are very good at prioritizing the right questions. Remember, there are always easier marks ahead, so never linger on a question!

Adjusting your Speed

Towards the end: Most test-takers find themselves needing to increase their speed towards the end of a subtest (around 2 or 3 sets left), so it's important to be very selective in the questions you attempt towards the end - you must flag, guess, and skip the time-consuming questions and discard without hesitation.

Behind at the halfway marker: If you're significantly behind - begin discarding, guessing, and skipping the time-consuming questions. If you're slightly behind, move quicker, and still consider skipping the harder questions.

Important Advice

- For each subtest, knowing the commonly tested question categories will help you differentiate between the more time-consuming questions and the easier questions.
- When doing mock exams under timed conditions - flag, guess, and skip.
- If you have to blindly guess, stick with one option (always pick A, etc.)
- Don't over-think questions. The students who over-think will be left with less time to spend on questions elsewhere. You must be merciless in your decisions, because unlike most school exams, time is the most important factor - it separates the weaker test-takers from the top scorers.

Discarding

Discarding is an important component in a strong approach to multiple-choice exams. For some subtests, such as Quantitative Reasoning and Verbal Reasoning, it plays a vital part of a good strategy.

Verbal Reasoning

For 'SBA Sets', you must discard each statement that doesn't agree with the question, and without any hesitation. The process of discarding for 'True-False Sets' is simpler and quicker: you only have three options (true/false/can't tell), and it's usually easier to discard 'True' or 'False'.

Quantitative Reasoning

It's usually quicker to locate the relevant data and solve for the answer, but sometimes discarding can be a useful tool for questions requiring little maths. For the more difficult and complex questions, there will be opportunities to rule out bold answers and guess when short on time, for example by estimating whether or not a percentage increase is more or less than 100%.

Abstract Reasoning

It's important to systematically discard patterns in your head. If you know a pattern has nothing to do with size (i.e. every shape is the same size), strike that off your mental checklist and move on to the next category (SSSPN).

Situational Judgement Test

Discarding can be used to remove half the options when picking a side, e.g. whether a response in appropriate or inappropriate, doubling your chance of getting the correct answer. This is easier for appropriateness questions than importance questions.

Subtest Difficulties

It's good to keep in mind the common challenges candidates face so you don't walk in making the same mistakes. You may have other weaknesses alongside these common problems - be sure to make a note of these when you find them so you can target these areas during your practice sessions.

Verbal Reasoning Difficulties

General

- Strict timing (2 minutes per passage).
- New 'Question Sets' forming the majority (four statements as options).
- Ambiguous information ('Can't Tell')
- Long and dense text.
- No keyword matches from statement/question.
- Difficult inferences.
- Deciding which questions to skip
- Selecting high yield keywords to skim for.
- Spotting qualifiers and absolutes in the passage/statement.
- Good pacing and adjusting for different questions.

What will slow me down?

- Trying to read the whole passage
- Questions with no keywords, or ineffective keywords.
- Overthinking answers.
- Hesitation when eliminating
- Harder inference questions (from two distinct areas in the passage, etc.)
- Misreading negative questions.
- Poor selection of keywords for skimming.

Decision Making Difficulties

General

- New subtest
- Use of critical thinking
- Use of data interpretation

Quantitative Reasoning Difficulties

General

- Strict timing (30 seconds per question).
- Complex multi-step questions.

- Familiarity with basic GCSE Maths.
- Checking the units for a calculation (conversions, etc.).
- Using mental maths/estimation for easier sets.
- Pacing and adjusting for different questions.
- Filtering and skipping harder questions.
- Use of the whiteboard.

What will slow me down?

- Questions which require more than two steps.
- Sets with complex diagrams/data - harder to locate relevant information.
- Using a calculator for simple calculations.

Abstract Reasoning Difficulties

General

- Strict time limit (1 minute per set).
- Attention-seekers.
- New Type 2, 3, and 4 Questions.
- Complex patterns.

What will slow me down?

- Not using a systematic approach (SSSPN).
- Not starting with the basic boxes.
- Conditional patterns.
- Multi-patterns.
- Number-shape patterns.

Situational Judgement Difficulties

General

- Final assessed subtest.
- Lengthy section
- Differences in scenario interpretation
- Not just based on common sense

What will slow me down?

- Not using a systematic approach
- Not reading the question carefully
- Overthinking the intricacies of each scenario

Practice

How to practice for the UCAT

There really isn't a shortcut when it comes to the UCAT, you must practice, but also be smart about it - there isn't much point repeating things you already do fairly well. Your practice sessions should be built around your weaknesses, as well as focusing on the common areas test-takers find hard.

Avoid doing the below at all costs:

- Mindlessly doing lots of questions and skimming the answers before finishing the session.
- Not timing yourself or putting yourself under any pressure during a practice session.
- Not reviewing mistakes properly and failing to identify weaknesses.
- Practicing whilst doing other things (watching TV, talking to someone on Facebook, etc.).
- Not using proven techniques and strategies - you're just doing your 'own thing'.

Here are some of the areas you're looking to improve:

- Strategic use of the timer and good adjustment of speed.
- Ability to quickly differentiate between the more time-consuming questions and easier questions.
- Honed discipline to move on when a question is taking too long.
- Efficient use of strategies to derive the correct answer.
- Good use of time-saving principles (utilizing mental maths, etc.).

After enough practice, and without much thought, you should be able to anticipate the common question types, quickly locate the relevant data (keywords in VR, numbers from a table, patterns in AR, etc.), and automatically apply a good method to get to the answer.

Mimic exam pressure

It's important to mimic the pressure you would feel in an exam situation. Don't just aim to 'solve' questions when you practice - we know you could do most of them if you had enough time. A lot of the strategies in this book won't work as well if you don't work on them under timed conditions: things like using the timer efficiently, discarding, keyword skimming, etc., are all there to help you save time, and so it wouldn't make sense nor would it be as effective to not practice under timed pressure.

Even if you're doing a single set by itself, time yourself using a stopwatch and note down where in the question you got up to as soon as it rings. You can then continue working on the set, but will also have an idea of how long it's taking over the recommended timing. This is especially important if you're doing a full mock exam or a series of sets: you will get into the habit of discarding ruthlessly and develop a discipline to move on from difficult questions, as well as completely skipping seemingly harder sets and coming back to them at the end if there's time. Doing all these things well and carefully managing your time heavily influences your final score - it's much more than just 'getting the question right'.

Using the computer

The UCAT, as you probably know, is not a pen and paper test. In order to better familiarize yourself with the test and under exam conditions, we recommend you practice as much as possible with online question banks and make the most of the mock exams available to you. A disadvantage of computerized testing is that there isn't a question paper you can mark or annotate - if you're used to circling information, or jotting down working next to questions, you may find this a bit harder. Do jot down the most important pieces of data onto your whiteboard, such as the intermediate solutions to a question, especially if you're overwhelmed with information.

This will be the on-screen calculator you'll be given on test-day:

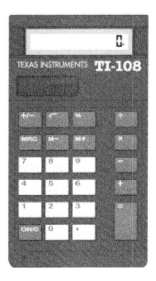

Keep track of your progress

- The whole point of practicing is to remove the bad habits which lead to poor performance, and to reinforce the habits which result in a good performance.
- Your UCAT success will be directly linked to how well you can identify your weaknesses.
- If you don't review your performance after every practice session (a mock exam, individual questions, etc.), you won't be able to improve as quickly.
- Keep some kind of log - it can be a notepad, your laptop (you can even use this course guide and annotate it).

Here are some useful questions to get you started:

1. What was my strongest section today?
2. What was my weakest section today?
3. What question types am I struggling with?
4. What question types slow me down? Why do they slow me down?
5. What question types do I find really easy?
6. What questions types can do I do really quickly?
7. Did I find any strategies hard to use or too slow?

Timeline of Skill Acquisition

Beginning of UCAT Study Period

- Familiarise yourself with recommended timings, question categories, and the basic approach for each subtest
- Recap some basic maths to get yourself upto speed
- Start noting down methods to help yourself save time in one place to aid your revision

Middle of UCAT Study Period

- Focus on individual subtests and questions one by one - start practicing under timed conditions
- Actively implement the strategies, techniques, and time saving principles from this course
- Develop a log of weaknesses and areas you want to work on more
- Do one mock exam per week and start getting comfortable using a whiteboard and the on screen calculator

End of UCAT Study Period

- Place a larger emphasis on computerised mock exams under strict time conditions
- Continue to log your performance after every session and take the time to carefully review each mistake.
- Question banks like ukcat.ninja and the practice papers on the UCAT website allow you to practice your skills and exam technique.

Practice Resources

Official Guide

Ensure you familiarize yourself with the official UCAT guide - it contains lots of important information and should be able to provide answers to any questions you may have. Also, take advantage of the good number of practice questions inside.

Official Practice Tests

You're only given two practice mock exams, so do the individual subtest practice questions first, and save the practice exams for when you're ready, and when you feel more prepared. You can rely on these questions being highly representative of the real exam, but you're only given a few, so try not waste them - do these questions under strict timing and in a quiet space.

Official tour

Recently, the UCAT consortium have provided some excellent resources to prepare candidates for test-day - the 'tour' that's available on the website will give you a good idea of how everything works (online calculator, scroll bar, etc.) and help you get comfortable with the general layout.

Official UCAT Practice App

Most people will have a bit of free time on the road, and that's where this application can come in handy: download this free app and run through the questions (although there aren't many).

Online Question Banks

Check out www.ukcat.ninja for a range of exam-style UCAT questions with detailed worked solutions and tutorials.

Verbal

Reasoning

What is 'Verbal Reasoning'?

This section tests your ability to both understand a piece of text and work out whether stated facts or conclusions match up to the passage. Importantly, you don't need to 'know' anything for this section. In fact, if you start incorporating your own knowledge, you may find yourself getting things wrong. You should only use information in the passages of text given to you to answer the questions.

Verbal reasoning isn't just testing your ability to read or even understand a piece of text - it primarily tests how well you can decide whether something is true, false or unsupported by evidence given. You'll be held accountable by patients and colleagues for everything you do, and it'll be helpful if you can make decisions based on sound reasoning that doesn't go beyond the evidence in front of you. Don't worry, most of you can reason perfectly well - however, this section is made extremely tough by its strict timing, but more on that later.

Why do we have to do VR?

Without question, reading and evaluating a wide range of written information will form a big part of your medical education and future career as a clinician, whatever you decide to go in to. Certainly, as a student, you'll come across many forms of information: textbooks, course material, Internet articles, case studies, journals, exam questions, and lecture slides. You will need to understand, digest, and scrutinize this information, as well as selecting the relevant areas as quickly as possible.

As medical information is becoming more readily available, there is a greater need to distinguish trustworthy sources and to carefully assess claims made. Moreover, later on as a clinician, you'll be continually working with novel medical research, and will have to evaluate and examine published articles in journals. Patients are frequently exposed to presumptuous, unreasonable, and sometimes extreme statements in health news and around the Internet. Consequently, it's imperative for doctors to question assumptions, identify poorly drawn conclusions, and spot unsound inferences - you'll become sick of these if you take the BMAT!

In the treatment of a patient, doctors must quickly sift through all the information directed towards them (on the Internet, from the patient themselves, from other doctors etc.), and must be careful not to make unreasonable assumptions. The VR exam requires you to work with a wide range of passages, and you should not consider any information or knowledge beyond the passage. You may also be expected to understand the difference between correlation and causation; it's essential to consider confounding factors before drawing any firm conclusions.

As a clinician, it probably won't come as a surprise that you will often need to select and evaluate information quickly and under pressure. When speaking to patients in a clinic, or when a patient is in a critical condition, there is limited time in which a doctor must make a diagnosis and draw upon the information given to him. Having strong reasoning skills, as well as being able to identify relevant information under pressure, is crucial. In a nutshell, this is what's being tested this subtest.

To be perfectly honest, we can talk until the cows come home about why we have to do VR, but at the end of the day, the most important answer is "because it's in the UCAT". This is the case for all five sections, but we've included a short "Why do we have to do this" at the start of each chapter just for fun.

The short answer is because the UCAT people tell you to. The long answer is that medical schools expect students to have a certain level of reasoning that is appropriate for the countless bits of text and journals you'll have to read all through your career as a doctor.

Numbers for this section

- **Time**

    22 minutes total = 1 minute for instructions + 21 minutes for questions
- **Questions**

    44 questions total

    11 passages (4 questions each)

    Two question types: True/False Sets and 'SBA' Sets

You have 21 minutes to do 44 questions, with a 1 minute break at the start. There are 11 passages of text, which means you have to do 4 questions per passage. You can work it out; that leaves 2 minutes per set of 4 questions or passage, which amounts to around 30 seconds per question. You're not alone if you feel horrified at those timings. In the strategy section, we'll give you all you need to know to be as efficient as possible and to stick to these timings.

Question Formats

In this section, there are two types of questions that you will come across. You know that you're given a passage accompanied by 4 questions, and this comprises a set. These can either be a 'Single Best Answer (SBA)' set or a 'True-False' set. These aren't the official names for these types of questions, but for ease of understanding, we'll just call them that.

Here is an example of a **'True-False' set:**

The London Underground is a railway system - also known as a rapid transit system - that serves a large part of Greater London, United Kingdom and some neighbouring areas. It is the world's oldest underground system. Services began on 10 January 1863 on the Metropolitan Railway; most of the initial route is now part of the Hammersmith & City line. Despite its name, about 55% of the network is above ground. Popular local names include the Underground and, more colloquially, the Tube, in reference to the cylindrical shape of the system's deep-bore tunnels.

The Underground has 276 stations and runs over 243 miles (408 km) of line, making it the longest underground railway in the world, and one of the most served in terms of stations. There are also numerous closed stations. In 2005 971 million passengers used the Underground and for the first time ever in 2007, over one billion passengers were recorded. As of March 2007, just over 3 million passengers use the Underground each day, with an average of 3.4 million passengers on weekdays.

Since 2003, the Underground has been part of Transport for London (TfL), which also administers numerous other transport-related functions, including the famous red double-decker buses. The former London Underground Limited was a subsidiary of London Regional Transport, a statutory corporation.

The first trains were steam-hauled, which required effective ventilation to the surface. Ventilation shafts at various points on the route allowed the engines to expel steam and bring fresh air into the tunnels. One such vent is at Leinster Gardens, W2. In order to preserve the visual characteristics in what is still a well-to-do street, a five-foot-thick (1.5 m) concrete façade was constructed to resemble a genuine house frontage.

1. **The London Underground is the oldest underground system in the world.**

   A. True
   B. False
   C. Can't Tell

2. It is estimated that the total passenger count on the Underground in a year will reach one billion, for the first time, in 2020.

A. True
B. False
C. Can't Tell

3. There are over 100 ventilation shafts along the Underground network.

A. True
B. False
C. Can't Tell

4. A greater proportion of the London Underground network is above ground than below ground.

A. True
B. False
C. Can't Tell

As you can see, you're given a passage of text alongside a question, which comprises a statement and a choice between true, false and can't tell as your answer. You'll consecutively have 4 of these questions to the same passage for a 'True-False' set.

Importantly, there are only around 3 True-False sets in the UCAT out of a total of 11 sets. The remaining questions are SBA sets.

Here is an example of an 'SBA' set:

Gorillas are ground-dwelling, predominantly herbivorous apes that inhabit the forests of central Africa. The eponymous genus Gorilla is divided into two species, the Eastern gorilla and the Western gorilla, and either four or five subspecies. They are the largest living primates by physical size. The DNA of gorillas is highly similar to that of humans, from 95-99% depending on what is counted, and they are the next closest living relatives to humans after the chimpanzees and bonobo.

Western mountain gorillas mostly eat foliage, such as leaves, stems, pith, and shoots, while fruit makes up a very small part of their diets. Mountain gorilla food is widely distributed and neither individuals nor groups have to compete with one another. As a result, they are not required to travel very far each day as they do not need to scavenge for food. Eastern lowland gorillas have more diverse diets, which vary seasonally.

Leaves and pith are commonly eaten, but fruits can make up as much as 25% of their diets. Since fruit is less available, lowland gorillas must travel long distances each day. Eastern gorillas will also consume termites, ants and aquatic herbs where available. Gorillas rarely drink water because the succulent vegetation they consume can be composed of up to 50% water.

Wild gorillas have relatively few predators. One possible predator is the leopard, although we lack conclusive evidence which proves that this is the case; gorilla remains have been found in leopard faeces, but this may be the result of scavenging. When a troop of gorillas is attacked by humans, leopards, or other gorillas, an individual silverback will protect the group, even at the cost of his own life. When confronted by danger, a silverback gorilla will often begin to charge before stopping short of the threat, a scare tactic known as the 'bluff charge'. Zoologist George Schaller has reported that "silverback gorilla and a leopard were both found dead from mutually inflicted wounds". Furthermore, a group of rangers in the Virunga National park have stated that they often observe leopards consuming gorilla carcasses.

1. **Which of the following is listed by the passage as being eaten by the Western gorilla but not by the Eastern gorilla?**

    A. Fruit
    B. Shoots
    C. Pith
    D. Termites

2. **According to the passage, which of the following is most likely to be false?**

A. The gorilla can be broken down to distinct species which can be further broken down into sub-species.

B. Silverback gorillas have been known to sacrifice themselves to protect their troop.

C. Gorillas do not typically need to drink water.

D. Silverback gorillas typically weigh twice as much as female gorillas.

3. **Which of the following considerations is not listed by the passage as supporting the theory that the leopard preys on the gorilla?**

A. Gorilla remains have been found in leopard faeces.

B. A gorilla and a leopard carcass have been found that show signs of a confrontation.

C. Anecdotal evidence offered by rangers.

D. Video footage showing a silverback 'bluff charging' an attacking leopard.

4. **According to the passage, which of the following statements is true?**

A. The gorilla and the human share upwards of 95% of their DNA.

B. Western gorillas must travel further each day to scavenge for food than the Eastern gorilla.

C. The gorilla is the closest living relative to humans.

D. Gorillas sleep in nests in the trees.

Again, this set contains a passage with a corresponding question. The difference, this time, is that you're given a question accompanied by 4 statements, of which only one is the correct answer. This is known as an SBA set, and you'll have 4 of these questions consecutively for a given passage. These form the vast majority of questions in VR, with 8 sets out of 11 being SBA sets, which amounts to 32 questions.

If you own an outdated UCAT book such as the 600Qs book, you won't find much information on the relatively new SBA sets. Be careful not to do too many True-False questions without practising the harder SBA sets that make up most of your VR exam.

Note: The solutions for both of these examples are at the end of this section - but we recommend you have another go after you've been through the strategy before you go anywhere near them!

Preparation Tips

1. **Always practice under timed conditions**

   For this section, you must be extremely strict with your timings in order to have a good chance of getting a high score, so you must practice under timed conditions. At first, it is ok to take as much time as you need to understand the different question types and learn how to implement the strategies that will ultimately make you more efficient and save you time. However, you must gradually increase your speed until you are able to do the questions under timed conditions. You don't want to develop a false sense of security by being lax with your practice sessions and not properly keeping to time. You will get the most out of the strategies by continuously applying them under pressure, and remember, the ultimate goal is to develop good habits, so you have less to worry about on test day.

2. **Be ruthless in discarding and selecting answers**

   Whenever you do VR sets, either a set at a time or part of a mock exam (always under timed conditions), you must be willing to discard questions and be confident when selecting your answer. We'll touch on this more later, but in terms of preparation, make a point of discarding answer options that might be wrong and just going for the correct answer, even if it's an educated guess. Likewise, discard entire questions that you know will take too much time or that you're spending too much time on (even if you're just doing a set of 4 questions). Students may lack a sense of urgency and ruthlessness when practising at home or during smaller practice sessions, but this is absolutely required if you want to have an edge on test day.

3. **Stick with an effective strategy**

   Don't play around with different strategies and end up mastering none of them. Stick with a solid strategy and keep employing it in your practice until it becomes second nature. Luckily for you, you don't need to worry about what strategy is best because we'll give you all of that in our later sections. We just want to implore you to stick with it and don't do your 'own thing' when you feel like it. That way, you'll have the best possible chance of getting a high VR score.

4. **Practice speed reading**

   You're going to have to go through relatively large amounts of text very quickly in this section, so you'll have an advantage if you're a fast reader. We don't teach you to read the passage in our strategy, but rather skim for keywords from the question or statement. Nonetheless, being able to skim and quickly digest information at the same time will be invaluable for this section. Look through our speed reading section and practice the technique with whatever you read on a daily basis - perhaps you might actually find it useful for many things beyond the UCAT!

True-False Sets

Approach

True-False Sets were originally the only verbal reasoning questions used in the UCAT; however they now only form around 3 of the 11 sets, with the rest being SBA Sets. You're given a set passage of text alongside four statements and you have to determine whether each one is True, False, or Can't Tell.

These sets are, without a doubt, much easier than the more involved SBA Sets because you only need to work with four statements in total, one for each question.

As with all sets in this section, there's a very specific approach you should follow and practice; the approach minimises the amount of time you waste on each question and becomes even more important in the later SBA sets.

Here's the **four-step approach** you should take for every True-False question:

1. Evaluate the Statement
2. Locate Keywords & Check the Context
3. Compare & Judge
4. Discard & Decide

When confronted with a True-False Set, it's imperative you don't read the passage first. To do so would be extremely time-consuming. It's much quicker instead for you to try skimming for high-yield keywords from the statement that lead you to the appropriate part of the passage. You'll end up understanding most of the passage anyway if you skim for keywords at the very beginning.

Here's the approach in more detail:

Step 1: Evaluate the Statement

For this first step, you must identify the most effective keyword(s) in the statement itself. For example, if the statement was: 'Strikes in the Ruhr slowed inflation', the best keywords would be 'Ruhr' and 'strikes'. The aim of the game is to select a keyword that will give you the highest chance of finding the appropriate part of the passage containing the answer. As a result, avoid keywords that are too broad and nonspecific. Here, 'inflation' would be a relatively nonspecific keyword to choose because there are references to 'inflation', 'hyperinflation', 'the exchange rate of the Mark against the US dollar' and the 'stability' of currency throughout the passage.

'Ruhr' is a slightly better keyword than 'strikes' because it is a proper noun, and the capitalisation makes it easier to skim for in the passage.

Always pick more than one keyword if you can to be safe, especially when the statement makes a comparison between two things. You can also pick a 'key phrase' if it makes more sense to skim for a sequence of words together, such as 'income tax' or 'exchange rate'.

You must also scrutinize the language: try to have a feel for the tone and boldness of the statement. For example, if the statement were: 'All workers in the Ruhr had their wages paid for by the German government when they went on general strike', we should note that this statement makes an absolute claim because of the usage of the word 'all'. It follows then that the passage must also be able to match this claim for it to be true. In this case, we cannot tell.

Step 2: Skim for Unique Keywords & Check the Context

Once you have your primary and secondary keyword, skim for them in the passage. Always be prepared to look for synonyms of the words you've chosen - but the more specific and unique the keyword, the more likely it'll appear.

Once you've found your keyword, read the entire sentence containing the word to make sure the context matches that of the statement. If you find the sentence or area of the passage you're reading isn't relevant to the statement given, then continue skimming for your keywords in the passage. It's possible that you'll come across your keyword several times before reaching the relevant part of the passage, and this is generally the case with more non-specific keywords, such as those that involve the topic of the passage in general.

The harder questions are usually those that either require a general inference from the passage or those that are unhelpfully broad in that they don't have many keywords for you to skim for - only attempt these if you are confident you have enough time. Importantly, you'll find it easier to locate the relevant parts of the passage you've done a few questions and have a better feeling for topics in different areas of the passage.

Step 3: Compare and Judge

Now you have the relevant part of the passage, and the sentence containing the keywords you're looking for, read it carefully and compare it to the statement given. Consider reading adjacent sentences to those containing the keywords because if more information is required to reach an answer. Apply the basic metrics for evaluating a statement and don't over-think (we will be discussing these basic metrics in the strategy tutorial). Be aware that for the harder questions you may have to make an inference from the passage.

Step 4: Discard and Decide

In the final step, you'll find yourself either discarding answer options you know are definitely wrong or deciding straightaway on a correct answer. It's generally easier to discard 'true' - for something to be true, you have to be sure the passage totally agrees with the statement. Deciding between false and can't tell can sometimes be more of a blurry choice, but whatever you do, always stick with the basics and decide without hesitation. Students that over-think in this section tend not to finish all the questions, and as a result, forfeit potentially easier marks at the end of the paper.

This 4-step approach is the fastest way of approaching true-false sets. Don't worry if you're a bit sluggish and slow to begin with - after a bit of practice, you'll know exactly what you need to do for each step. In the strategy tutorial, we go over how to effectively choose the best keywords, as well as the basic metrics you should apply when trying to decide if something is true, false or can't tell.

Key Reminders:

1. **Don't read the passage first.** If you do so, you're unlikely to finish the set in under 2 minutes.
2. **Don't assume that the first time you find the keyword in the passage, it is in the right context.** Move swiftly to skim further in the passage if the context is wrong and be prepared to repeat this several times.
3. Remember that the UKCAT interface allows you to **'flag' questions to come back to later** if you are unsure about whether or not you have time to do difficult questions.

Walkthrough

We're going to talk you through the 4-step approach by applying it to a question.

Here's the passage:

In recent years, there has been an increase in the number of heart transplantations to the point where demand significantly exceeds any reasonable expectation of the routine "supply" of suitable hearts from cadavers. By definition, patients who would benefit from heart transplantation are critically ill. Hence the limitation in supply inevitably means that some people will die before a suitable organ becomes available. This suggests an ethical motive for research into the application of xenografting to this issue.

Genetic manipulation is a possible way of preventing the hyperacute response whereby human antibodies act rapidly to reject the transplanted tissue as though responding to an infection. Current research is attempting to transfer the gene which directs the production of regulatory factors for human "complement" into pigs, so that the heart is no longer recognized as foreign. Conventional drug therapy is, however, still required to prevent rejection via binding to histocompatibility complexes, which react to the different tissue surface chemicals of an organ transplanted even within the same species. The actual technique being developed involves a single gene (it is presumed without a regulator).

There appear to be several groups of people working on this technique, and different groups appear to have chosen different genes to work with. A group from Cambridge was still some way from applying the technology to human recipients. In early 1995, they were only at the stage of producing homozygous lines of transgenic pigs. Other groups have progressed further with this genetic engineering, but none are at the stage of running clinical trials.

Question 1. The increase in the number of heart transplantations is due to an increasing number of people adopting unhealthy lifestyles.
A. True
B. False
C. Can't Tell

The first step is to **evaluate the statement**. This statement draws a comparison, specifically between 'heart transplantation' and people adopting 'unhealthy lifestyles'. The best keywords or phrases in this statement should be unique and specific to the statement - and so 'heart transplantation' and 'unhealthy lifestyle' are good choices. Less useful keywords to choose are those that are more non-specific, such as 'number' or 'adopt'.

Skimming for 'heart transplantation' and 'unhealthy lifestyle' in the passage, we find 'heart transplantation' mentioned straightaway in the first sentence. Reading the sentence, we find that it's in the wrong context and not relevant to our statement. We should then continue to skim further in the passage for our keywords. We find 'heart transplantation' mentioned a bit later on in the first paragraph. Reading the containing sentence, we find that, again, the context is wrong. The statement makes a direct comparison, but there's no mention of 'unhealthy lifestyles' anywhere in the first paragraph - we should be expecting to see it close to the keyword 'heart transplantation'. In fact, skimming for 'unhealthy lifestyle' in the passage reveals it isn't mentioned at all.

More information is required to be able to determine if this statement is true or false: there's no mention of people adopting unhealthy lifestyles anywhere in the passage, let alone a link to heart transplantation. The answer to this question is therefore 'Can't Tell'. As a result, we can decide on this as the correct answer and move swiftly onto the next question.

Question 2: A problem in heart transplantation is the host antibody response to the transplanted tissue.
A. True
B. False
C. Can't Tell

Again, **evaluating the statement**, the best keyword would be 'antibody response' because it's unique - it shouldn't appear many times in the passage and will, therefore, lead us to hopefully to the appropriate area. We already know that 'heart transplantation' appears twice in the first paragraph, so a more suitable second keyword would be 'tissue'.

Skimming for these keywords, we're led to the first sentence of the second paragraph, which contains both the keyword 'antibodies' and 'tissue' - indeed, reading the sentence, it's clear that the context is correct.

We should then **compare and judge** between what is said in the passage and the statement given, and see if they agree, contradict or can't be compared without more information. On comparison, the passage states how human antibodies 'act rapidly to reject the transplanted tissue' and so is consistent with our statement - this 'rejection' is clearly a problem in heart transplantation.

As a result, we should **decide** on 'True' being the correct answer without hesitation and move on to the next question.

Question 3: In 1995, a group from Cambridge were able to test genetic manipulation technology on human recipients.

A. True

B. False

C. Can't Tell

Upon **evaluating the statement**, we can see that '1995' is easily skimmed for in the passage. Alongside that, we should also skim for 'Cambridge' because it's also rather specific and a capitalized noun. When we **skim** for these keywords, we find both of these words in the final paragraph. Reading the two sentences containing these key elements, we know that we're in the right place and the **context** is correct. **Comparing** between the statement and passage, it's obvious what the answer is: there's a direct contradiction - the passage tells us that a 'group from Cambridge', in '1995', were 'still some way from applying the technology to human recipients', whereas the statement claims the opposite to be true. We can therefore confidently decide on 'False' as being the correct answer.

Question 4: Drug therapy is currently used to minimize rejection of a transplanted heart by the host.

A. True

B. False

C. Can't Tell

You should have an idea of the approach by now - we first start by **evaluating the statement** and picking out the best keywords, in this case probably 'Drug Therapy' together with 'Rejection'. We then **skim** for these keywords in the passage, which leads us nicely to the second paragraph, where both words are mentioned. Reading and **checking the context** confirms it's just what we're looking for with regards to our statement. The passage tells us that 'conventional drug therapy' is 'still required to prevent rejection... of an organ'. Upon **comparing** with the statement given, we can see that they agree with one another - the answer is therefore 'True'. **Decide** on this as your correct answer.

SBA Sets

Approach

The majority of questions you'll come across in the verbal reasoning section will be SBA sets - around 8 out of the 11 sets. Unfortunately, these sets are more difficult than their True-False counterparts. The difficulty lies in the increased amount of work you have to do to and the little time you have in which to do it. Therefore, it is even more important to adopt a solid approach that is as time efficient as possible.

If you remember, for True-False sets you're given a statement and have to evaluate whether it's True, False or Can't Tell with respect to the passage. For SBA sets, you're given a question and then four statement options, of which you have to pick the one that is correct.

The approach to SBA sets is largely similar to what you would do for True-False sets, with a few additions- importantly though, skimming the passage for high-yield keywords is crucial.

Here's the **five-step approach** you should take for every SBA set:

1. Assess the Question
2. Evaluate the Statement
3. Locate Keywords & Check the Context
4. Compare & Judge
5. Discard & Decide

Approach each statement in each SBA question as you would for a True-False statement, and be prepared to do lots of discarding until you get to the correct statement. If you reach step 5, discard the statement and still have not decided on an answer, you will have to return to step 2 and repeat with the subsequent statement. You're probably wondering how on earth you can get through an SBA set properly with so little time - but that's where discarding comes in: you only need to evaluate a maximum of three statements for each SBA question because once you've discarded the first three, the fourth statement must be your answer. Even better, if you can decide confidently that the first statement is the correct answer, you can discard the remaining three statement options and save yourself a lot of time. All these little ways of saving time come together and make it possible to actually finish an SBA set, but only if you stick with the approach and don't overthink things.

Here's the approach in more detail:

Step 1: Assess the Question

This is the only step you don't have for the True-False sets. There is a limited range of question types that they could ask you and they are more or less as follows:

1. Questions containing keywords: 'Which of the following is not a counter-insurgency method listed in the passage?'
2. Which of the following is most likely to be true?
3. Which of the following is most likely to be false?
4. Which of the following is least likely/unlikely to be true?
5. Which of the following cannot be true?
6. Which of the following can be inferred from the passage/a conclusion from the passage?

Although the wording will vary, the majority of questions that are asked will fall into one of the above categories. Put simply, a question can only require you to find the statement that is either true, false or can't tell, or one that makes a correct or incorrect inference from the passage, or one that draws/does not draw a correct conclusion from the passage.

Assessing the question is important because it'll inform what you're looking for, and students can easily go wrong here if they're not careful and pushed for time. In particular, it can be surprisingly easy to forget what the question actually wants when you're evaluating the statements: if the question wants a statement that is false, don't fall into the trap of selecting a true statement as the answer; as stupid as it sounds, in the heat of the moment you may see a true statement and think it's what you're looking for.

Something that you may find helpful is if you make a checklist table on your whiteboard during the instructions period:

Q	T	F	CT
1	✓		
2		✓	
3		✓	✓

Students who make such a table find it to be an easy reference for what the question wants when evaluating statements. It's certainly something helpful to fall back on if you're under a lot of pressure.

Another important point is that you need to be careful in what you can and can't discard with regards to the question. If the question is looking for something that is 'least likely to be true', then the correct statement could either 'false' or 'can't tell', and so you can only discard 'true' statements. On the other hand, if the question wanted something that 'cannot be true', you can discard both 'true' and 'can't tell' statements.

The hardest questions will be those that require you to draw an inference or conclusion. Don't get too hung up on these. To keep to time, you may need to 'flag' and skip them to come back to later. Approach questions that have no keywords (those that want something that is 'likely true', etc.) by evaluating each statement in the same way you do for True-False sets. Note that questions that ask for a statement the author would 'agree' with could either be something that is clearly a 'true' statement or something that requires an inference.

An Aside: Keyword Questions

'For what reason might one want to place a kiln in a trench rather than on the surface of the ground?'

The relatively easier questions are those that contain helpful keywords in the question because they help us locate the appropriate part of the passage early on. With these keyword questions, select helpful keywords to skim for in the passage as you would if you were approaching a statement - you could then skim for these keywords before evaluating the first statement because it will hopefully lead you to a paragraph that contains all you need to know to select the best statement option. If the question contains relatively weaker keywords, then it may be more helpful to skim either for keywords from just the statements themselves, or keywords from both the first statement and the question.

As an example, for the sample question above, we could skim for 'trench' and 'kiln', which could lead us to the most appropriate part of the passage. With practice, you'll have a better feeling for what to skim for and when.

Step 2: Evaluate the Statement

This step is essentially the same as that for True-False sets. For each statement consider the language, and importantly, skim for high-yield keywords to locate the relevant part of the passage (if you haven't done so already for a question containing keywords).

Step 3: Locate Keywords & Check the Context

Once you have your keywords (either from the question or your statement), skim for them in the passage and check the context, making sure it matches what the question is looking for or what the statement is claiming. You may need to read adjacent sentences.

Step 4: Compare & Judge

Having located the right part of the passage, compare it to the statements given, starting with the first. Apply your basic metrics - whether the statement is True, False or Can't Tell, or a valid inference - and don't overthink.

Step 5: Discard & Decide

If you're confident the first statement is the correct answer, then it's imperative you make this decision and discard the rest without even reading them. This is the one of the few ways you can save time. If the first statement is incorrect, discard it and evaluate the next statement, going through the same process again.

Remember, you should only be evaluating a maximum of three statements, because once you've done three, the final statement should be the correct answer. Some courage is needed here - you won't always feel confident in deciding on an answer or discarding something, but, feelings aside, you haven't got time to be going through things twice or 'playing it safe': don't overthink, and there are always easier marks up ahead.

There are certainly questions you'll find you have to skip, and it's best to not hung up on these; even better, with practice, you should be able to spot the questions that aren't even worth attempting in order to save time.

Key Reminders:

1. **Carefully assess the question** because it informs what you're looking for when evaluating statements.
2. **Be ruthless in discarding**. Discarding without hesitation and deciding confidently will count greatly when it comes to saving time and finishing the test.

Walkthrough

We're going to talk you through the 5-step approach by applying it to a question.

Here's the passage:

Acetic acid is an organic compound with the chemical formula CH_3COOH. It is a colourless liquid that when undiluted is also called glacial acetic acid. Vinegar is roughly 3-9% acetic acid by volume, making acetic acid the main component of vinegar apart from water. Acetic acid has a distinctive sour taste and pungent smell. Although it is classified as a weak acid, concentrated acetic acid is corrosive and can attack the skin.

Acetic acid is the second simplest carboxylic acid (after formic acid). It is simply two small structural groups, an acetyl group and a hydroxyl group, linked (AcOH). It is an important chemical reagent and industrial chemical, mainly used in the production of cellulose acetate for photographic film and polyvinyl acetate for wood glue. In households, diluted acetic acid is often used in descaling agents. In the food industry, acetic acid is used under the food additive code E260 as an acidity regulator and as a condiment.

Acetic acid is a strong eye, skin, and mucous membrane irritant. Prolonged skin contact with acetic acid may result in tissue destruction, although the blisters that will form might not appear until hours after exposure. Inhalation exposure to acetic acid vapours at 10 ppm could produce some irritation of eyes, nose, and throat; at 100 ppm marked lung irritation and possible damage to lungs, eyes, and skin might result. Vapour concentrations of 1,000 ppm cause marked irritation of eyes, nose and upper respiratory tract and cannot be tolerated. These predictions were based on animal experiments and industrial exposure. Skin sensitization to acetic acid is rare but has occurred. Latex gloves offer no protection, so special resistant gloves, such as those made of nitrile rubber, are worn when handling the compound. Concentrated acetic acid can be ignited with difficulty in the laboratory. It becomes a flammable risk if the ambient temperature exceeds 39 °C (102 °F) and can form explosive mixtures with air above this temperature (explosive limits: 5.4-16%).

Question 1: Which of the following is not listed in the passage as a potential use of acetic acid?

A. Use in the production of vinegar.
B. Use in the production of synthetic fibres.
C. Use in the production of wood glue.
D. Use as a descaling agent.

The first step is to **assess the question**. The question is looking for a statement that's either 'false' or 'can't tell'. We can discard statements that are 'true'. For this question, we're given some keywords, more specifically 'acetic acid'. However, we have to be careful here because a cursory glance at the passage tells us that the topic is acetic acid, so it's likely it'll appear quite a few times. Bearing this in mind, we should also pick a keyword to skim for when **evaluating** the first statement - 'vinegar' is good for the job.

Skimming for both 'vinegar' and 'acetic acid', we're led to the second sentence of the first paragraph. **Comparing** between the passage and the statement with reference to what the question wants (a statement not listed as a potential use of acetic acid), we're told that 'acetic acid is the main component of vinegar apart from water' and so we know the first statement is true. **Discard** (a), because it's not what the question is looking for and therefore incorrect.

Repeating the same process again for the second statement, upon **evaluation**, it's clear that 'synthetic fibres' are the best keywords. **Skimming** for these in the passage, we find that they don't appear anywhere in the passage. A rule of thumb is that if something obvious and important, such as a unique keyword, doesn't appear anywhere, it's most likely 'can't tell'. There's nothing in the passage we can use to **compare** to the statement, and the answer lies beyond the scope of the passage. This answer is therefore correct. At this point, we **decide** on (b) as the correct answer and discard the remaining two statements without even looking at them. We swiftly move on to the next question.

Question 2: According to the information in the passage, which of the following statements is most likely false?
A. Blisters that form as a result of skin contact with acetic acid will not form for many hours.
B. Acetic acid has a strong, sharp smell.
C. Acetic acid is the most common acid that is used in the food condiment industry.
D. Acetic acid could form an explosive mixture with air at a temperature of 60°C.

Assessing the question, we find no keywords, and we're asked to find the statement that's true. We should approach each statement as we would for a true-false set until we get to the correct answer. **Evaluating** the first statement, we find that good keywords for skim for are 'blisters' alongside 'acetic acid'. **Skimming** for both of these words, we find them in second sentence of the final paragraph, and they're in the right context. Reading the sentence containing the keywords and **comparing** it to the passage reveals a direct agreement: both state that blisters, as a result of 'skin contact with acetic acid' will not appear 'until hours' after exposure. This is a simple rewording of the passage by the statement. This statement is therefore correct because the question is looking for a 'true' statement - **decide** on this as the correct answer and, importantly, **discard** the remaining three statement options in order to save valuable time. This is a relatively easier question, and they do exist - use these to maximise time on the harder questions.

Question 3: Which of the following is not listed as a risk associated with the inhalation of acetic acid vapour of 100ppm?

A. Irritation of the eyes.
B. Damage to the skin.
C. Damage to the lungs.
D. Irritation to the upper respiratory tract.

Upon **assessing this question**, we can tell straight away that there are a few high-yield keywords we can use - the most obvious one being '100 ppm', while also keeping 'inhalation' as a second keyword. Importantly, the question is looking for something that's either 'false' or 'can't tell'. We can discard anything that's 'true'.

The keywords in this question are good enough that we can **skim** straight for them in the passage without looking at the statements. While skimming for '100 ppm', bear in mind that we're looking for any number with the unit ppm, and not necessarily an exact match. Indeed, this leads us to the third sentence of the final paragraph, as well as a few adjacent sentences. Checking the **context**, we know that we're in the right place as indicated by the mention of 'inhalation exposure' in the passage. We should then proceed to reading the whole sentence and adjacent sentences carefully; the passage lists several risks associated with inhalation of vapours of acetic acid, but at 100 ppm specifically, it tells us that 'possible damage to lungs, eyes, and skin might result'. As a result, we can **discard** (c), (a) and (b) in one swoop, which means (d) must be the correct answer. Indeed, 'irritation to the upper respiratory tract' is listed under 1000 ppm. We can therefore **decide** on (d) and move on to the final question.

Question 4: From the information given in the passage, which of the following statements is true?

A. Latex gloves should be worn when handling acetic acid, as nitrile rubber gloves are inadequate.
B. Formic acid is structurally the least complex carboxylic acid,
C. The main component of vinegar is acetic acid.
D. All methods of producing photographic film require the use of acetic acid.

The final question offers no keywords, and **assessing** it is simple - we need to find a 'true' statement. **Evaluating** the first statement, the best keywords would be 'latex' and 'nitrile rubber'. **Skimming** for these keywords, they appear near the end of the final paragraph, and reading it carefully confirms it's in the right **context**. The passage tells us that 'latex gloves offer no protection' and 'those made of nitrile rubber are worn' when handling acetic acid: upon **comparison**, this is a direct contraction to the statement. Discard (a) and continue by **evaluating** the second statement. The best keywords for the second statement are 'formic acid' and 'carboxylic acid'. Indeed, these lead us to the first sentence of the second paragraph, which essentially tells us that 'formic acid' is the 'simplest carboxylic acid'; the passage then goes on to describe the structural groups of acetic acid. From this, it's reasonable to infer that formic acid is the least complex carboxylic acid, at least structurally - and therefore (b) is the correct answer. **Decide** on this option and **discard** the remaining two statements in order to save valuable time.

Strategy

Timing

When it comes to anything in the UKCAT, getting to grips with the timing is essential - and make sure you don't just know how much time you have, but understand how best make the use of this time.

Here's a reminder of how much time you have for VR:

1 minute	Instructions
21 minutes	44 questions (11 sets)

If we break it down further, we get the following:

<2 minutes	Time per set (4 questions)
<30 seconds	Time per question

If we divided each set of 4 questions equally by the amount of time given, we're left with just under 2 minutes per set. It then follows that we have less than 30 seconds for each question.

We have to warn you, it's unlikely you're going to be able to keep under 2 minutes for every set, especially not the SBA sets. You should aim to finish the True-False sets as quickly as possible, preferably under 1 minute 40 seconds - but don't rush so much you start making mistakes.

Checking the timer

Just in case you didn't know, there's a timer at the top right hand corner of the screen, and it starts counting down from 21 minutes as soon as you start. People check the timer in different ways. Some prefer checking it after every passage (to make sure they haven't gone over 2 minutes), helping them strictly keep to the alloted time. For many though, this can be slightly distracting, especially when you're under a lot of pressure.

Ideally, you should be able to have a rough feeling of how long you're spending on each set or if you're going over 2 minutes without even looking at the timer, and this is only possible after lots of timed practice. What would be useful if this is the case, then, is having a halfway marker; this is a recommended time remaining you should aim for at the beginning of the 6th set, which gives you a good indication of how fast or slow you're going and whether you need to speed up for the second half of the section.

The time remaining for the halfway marker is as follows: **12 minutes remaining**

This gives you a good indication of how fast or slow you're going and whether you need to speed up for the second half of the section. If you're behind at the halfway marker, the best strategy is to begin flagging, guessing, and skipping the more complex questions.

Important advice

- With the little flexibility you have for VR, don't be too surprised if you don't have much (if any) time to review answers or questions.
- Make sure you always select an answer, even if it's a blind guess.
- Remember, although you have relatively little time for each question, you should be able to save some time on the easier questions, and hopefully leave more time for the harder passages.
- When you practice, try to focus on the harder SBA Sets; these will comprise the majority of the marks and will be much more time consuming in comparison to True-False Sets.

Saving time

You should always be on the lookout for opportunities to save time throughout the UCAT, and this should definitely be the case for verbal reasoning. We've come up with a few ways we think will save you time in this section:

1. **Don't read the passage first**. As you already know, this is unnecessarily time-consuming. You can get the information you need more quickly by skimming for keywords.
2. **Get good at choosing high-yield keywords**. The purpose of choosing a keyword is for it to guide you to the part of the passage relevant to the question. The better you are at weeding out poor keywords and selecting those that are both easy to spot and highly specific, the more time you'll save.
3. **Don't overthink**. It's so easy to get hung up on whether something is False or Can't Tell, or if you're missing something in the passage: whatever it is, you haven't got the time to sit around - just put decide on an answer confidently having applied the basic metrics.
4. **Discard without hesitation**. This is similar to not overthinking, but the importance of discarding, especially in SBA sets, cannot be overemphasised. Discard statements without hesitation until you get to the correct statement, and if, for example, you're relatively confident that the first SBA statement is correct, then discard the remaining three without even looking at them.
5. **Avoid difficult questions**. The harder questions are those that look for an inference, want you to draw a conclusion, or contain very few high-yield keywords you can actually work with. You'll know what's hard and what's not with practice, but sometimes it's more efficient to not even attempt these questions and come back to them at the end if you have time. This is certainly what you should be doing if you find yourself behind schedule.
6. **Learn to speed read**. Most of us can't speed read, but, without stating the obvious too much, it's a useful skill to have. You may as well pick it up and it'll stay with you for life. There are

quite a few good applications and resources out there that can help you get better and those are all mentioned in our skills section.

Remember, time equals marks in the UCAT. The aim of the game is to maximise the amount of time you have for the questions you're most likely to get right. To do so, you must be able move quickly and avoid the questions you probably won't get right with the time given.

Identifying Keywords

Keywords form a core part of the approach. They help us target the relevant parts of the passage quickly, without having to read the entire passage. There are two good qualities of a high-yield keyword: they are easy to spot, and they are specific to a certain part of the passage.

Specific keywords

Take a look at this statement:

'Women took part in all of the Ancient Olympic games.'

Within a given statement (or question as for some SBA sets), there will likely be more than one potential keyword you could use. In this case, there are two keywords or phrases we can skim for, that is 'women' and 'Ancient Olympic games'. We should always be aware of the topic of the passage - if the entire passage is on the topic of the Ancient Olympic games, then skimming for it alone as a keyword would be time-consuming because it'll probably appear several times in the wrong context. Sometimes this is unavoidable, and you'll just have to continuously skim and check the context, and then continue skimming if it doesn't match.

A better keyword in this case would be 'women' as it's relatively important to the statement and unlikely to appear multiple times in the passage. Nonetheless, in this situation, we should skim for both keywords together - always have a secondary keyword, if you can, when evaluating statements, and this is especially important when two things are being compared:

'Water can be more dangerous than alcohol if used wrongly.'

It's certainly not difficult skimming for two keywords at once, and we encourage you to always do so just in case one keyword fails to deliver.

Easy-to-spot keywords

There are a handful of keywords that you should always go for if you see them, and they tend to be those that are super easy to find the passage. Always consider skimming for:

1. Acronyms: *'HTTP is often used to access the internet.'*
2. Capitalised nouns: *'The World Wide Web was central to the development of the information age.'*
3. People: *'Berners-Lee had a vision of a global hyperlinked information system.'*
4. Dates: *'The United Nations were formed in 1927.'*
5. Numbers: *'Most stars reach temperatures of over 1 million Kelvin.'*

On more rare occasions, there may be no helpful keywords in a statement whatsoever: do consider skipping these and definitely if you're short on time.

True, False or Can't Tell

When comparing between the passage and a given statement, always apply the basic metrics to decide whether something is true, false or can't tell:

True	Agree
False	Contradict
Can't tell	Beyond
Not sure?	Probably 'Can't tell'

Just ask yourself these three simple questions: Does the passage agree with the statement? If not, is the statement directly contradicting the passage? Do I need outside information, or information beyond the passage, to fully compare the statement with the passage?

Some questions can be slightly ambiguous, but you should always be able to discard at least one of true, false or can't tell if you ask these simple questions. Always stick with the basics and avoid overthinking things. For many questions, if you're unsure of the answer, there's a good chance it's 'can't tell'; you need to be certain the passage agrees or contradicts with the statement before you can decide it's true or false.

Further illustration of the anatomy of true, false and can't tell statements can helpfully breakdown the common ways questions are written.

True statements

A true statement typically:

1. Rewords the passage
2. Draws a valid inference from the passage
3. Occasionally works with numbers

For example:

'In Ancient Greece, only free, land owning, native-born men could be citizens entitled to the full protection of the law in a city-state.'

    1. Correct rewording:

'To be entitled to the full protection of the law in a city state, a man must have been born in the city, be free, and possess land.'

The statement won't repeat the same sentence from the passage word for word, but rather reword it whilst retaining the meaning. These are common and should be relatively easy to get right.

2. Correct inference:

'In comparison to free citizens, slaves weren't entitled to full protection.'

Inferences are more difficult because they won't always be obvious and requires you to take the information in the passage a step further - you'll need to make a logically sound and reasonable conclusion with only the information given in the passage. It's very important you don't bring in personal outside information to answer to draw an inference.

False statements

A false statement typically:

1. Wrongly rewords and uses antonyms
2. Changes or adds a qualifier or absolute

For example:

'In Ancient Greece, only free, land owning, native-born men could be citizens entitled to the full protection of the law in a city-state. Slaves had no power or status, but some had the right to have a family and own property.'

1. Incorrect rewording:

'Slaves had the right to have a family, but not own property'

A statement can misquote and/or wrongly insert antonyms into a sentence leading it to contradict the passage and therefore making it false.

2. Changing a qualifier or absolute:

'Slaves had some power.'

'All slaves were allowed to have a family.'

A statement can twist the meaning of the passage by simply changing and adding a qualified or absolute word. For example, the passage states that 'slaves had no power', where 'no' makes the sentence absolute; the statement, however, claims that 'slaves had some power', with 'some' being a qualified word. Similarly, the passage tells us that 'some [slaves] had the right to have a family', whereas the false statement claims that 'all slaves were allowed to have a family'. There's a somewhat subtle switch here in usage of qualified and absolute words between the sentence and passage, and this can easily render a statement false. This is a UCAT favourite, so keep a lookout for these shifts.

Can't tell statements

A can't tell statement typically:

1. Contains information not mentioned the passage
2. Makes an unsupported comparison in the passage
3. Makes an unsupported absolute claim
4. Contains an inference that is unsupported by the passage

For example:

'In Ancient Greece, only free, land owning, native-born men could be citizens entitled to the full protection of the law in a city-state. Slaves had no power or status, but some had the right to have a family and own property. Foreigners paying a large sum of money were able to secure property.'

1. Missing information:

'Women could not own land.'

Commonly, statements bring in extra information beyond the passage; generally, if we're unable to find important keywords or related synonyms in the passage, there's a good chance the statement is can't tell. In this example, there's no mention of 'women', so we can't really judge whether this statement is true or false.

2. Unsupported comparison:

'Slaves must have owned more property than foreigners.'

Two unrelated pieces of information from the passage may be used in a statement and compared; again, we always need more information to be able to say whether such comparisons are true or false, and so 'can't tell' is the most appropriate option in these situations. In this example, we don't have enough information from the passage to say whether this statement is true or not.

3. Unsupported absolute claim:

'Foreigners are always able to secure property as long as they pay a large sum of money.'

Similar to qualifier-absolute shifts employed in false statements, a can't tell statement can make absolute something in the passage that hasn't been qualified. For example, we know that 'foreigners paying a large sum of money are able to secure property', but we don't know if this is 'always' the case as the statement claims. The statement certainly isn't agreeing with the passage, but it isn't directly contradicting it either. As a result, we need more information to be able to comment on this statement - and so, by definition, this is 'can't tell'.

4. Unsupported inference:

'As slaves had no status or power, they were mistreated by those with power and status.'

An unsupported inference is one that requires outside knowledge to answer; outside knowledge means anything that you've learnt in your school curriculum or from books, for example. What doesn't count as outside knowledge are obvious things that almost everyone should know (a submarine is a mode of underwater transportation, etc.) and whatever is in the passage. In this case, you may know that there's been a long history of slaves being mistreated from your lessons at school or even that it was definitely the case in Ancient Greece, but we can't be certain that was the case without more information outside the passage.

Qualifiers & Absolutes

In VR, there's commonly a shift between qualified and absolute modifiers from the statement to the passage. Qualification of a sentence makes it less bold and open to different possibilities or events - for example: 'Lawrence can become a famous footballer, but long-term smoking may impair his performance'. In this example statement, 'can' and 'may' are qualifiers. Contrast this to a sentence that's absolute: 'Smoking will impair Lawrence's performance'. One way of differentiating absolute from qualified statements is to ask yourself if it sounds bold (likely absolute) or safe (generally qualified). Always scrutinize the language in both the statement and passage when comparing, making sure the modifiers match.

Familiarize yourself with the commonly used 'absolute' and 'qualified' modifiers:

Absolute	Qualified
All/Every	Most, many, numerous, a majority 'Many/numerous': does not necessarily suggest a majority. It simply refers to a large number of occurrences. 'Most/a majority': refers to more than 50% and reflects a large proportion of a population.
None/no	Not many, a small number, a minority, hardly any 'Not many, a small number', 'hardly any': represents a small number of occurrences. 'A minority': refers to a small proportion of occurrences.
Always	Commonly, usually, repeatedly Suggests a common occurrence (that doesn't 'always' happen) - it can be expected to occur in the majority of cases (above 50%).
Never	Rarely, infrequently, seldom Low probability of occurrence, but sometimes can occur.
Impossible	Unlikely, improbable Reflects a low probability of occurrence, but not impossible.
Certainly	Usually, probably Reflects a high probability of occurrence, but not a certain occurrence.

Speed Skimming

There's a difference between speed reading and speed skimming. There are lots of systems and platforms out there that claim to teach you how to speed read, but reading faster than a certain speed is always at the expense of comprehension. Most people read at a speed of 100 to 200 words per minute and evidence suggests that there is generally reduced comprehension when attempting to read faster than 300 words per minute. In short, speed reading anything you want to understand is probably a bad idea.

For the UKCAT, our strategy is rooted in finding high-yield keywords from the statement in the passage, and then closely scrutinizing the correct part of the passage, carefully reading the relevant sentences. Speed skimming, then, is important, and something you should definitely practice and hone in order to save time. To find your top reading speed, grab a book and move the pen across the page quicker and quicker until you can't read any faster. Your optimum reading speed will be a bit slower than this top speed.

Here are are three tips to increase your skimming speed:

1. Read selectively

When skimming a passage, try skimming past smaller connecting words such as 'and', 'I', 'am', 'but', 'because', 'as', etc. As a rule of thumb, just skim over words that are three letters or less. Here's an example paragraph with only the words you should be skim reading in bold:

My **fiancée** is an **avid listener** and **lover** of anything to do with **economics**. She **studied economics** at **Leeds University**, and since **graduating**, she has been **teaching economics** at the **local grammar school**. Her **favourite** area is **microeconomics** - the **theory** of **supply** and **demand** always gets her going.

2. Use a pointer

Even in the UCAT, you can use a pen to help you skim across the screen (as long as it's not touch screen). If not, you could use your finger as a pointer instead. Following pointer has been shown to increase reading speed because it forces you to skim efficiently and not reread things.

3. Move further back

Positioning yourself slightly further away from the screen may help you read more quickly - your field of vision enlarges with distance. If you find yourself skimming a bit too slowly, try moving back a few inches and see if it that makes a difference. When doing VR, actively remind yourself to shift further back, and certainly don't get into the bad habit of hunching over the screen. Do try to find your own optimal distance from the screen before test-day.

Summary

1. Questions that reword and contradict the passage

- The simplest questions (for both True-False Sets and SBA Sets) are statements which reword or contradict part of the passage.
- These questions are usually obvious and make for quick marks.

Important Advice

- Often keywords appear more than once in a passage, so continue skimming if the context doesn't match.
- If no keywords appear in the passage, there's a high chance it's Can't tell.

2. Statements that make an inference from the passage

- The more difficult statements are ones which draw a conclusion or inference from information in the passage.
- If you were to put such a conclusion or inference at the end, it should be logically sound, reasonable, and would be a sensible interpretation based on the preceding information.
- Remember, don't bring in any information from beyond the passage - if the passage does not support the assumptions made in a statement, the answer is 'Can't tell'.

If the inference is:

- True = LOGICALLY FOLLOWS
- False = CONTRADICTS
- Can't Tell = BEYOND

Important advice

- If you can't find a keyword, it's usually safe to go with 'Can't tell', but sometimes there may not be an obvious keyword or synonym you can skim for. You shouldn't linger on these questions - consider skipping them if you can.
- Some questions will need you to compare different parts of the passage, and this can be very time consuming. Discard, guess, and skip if you're short on time.

3. Manipulation of Qualifiers and Absolutes

- Don't always expect the statement to reword sentences in the passage - often there will be a subtle change in language that catches people out.
- A change from an 'absolute statement' to a 'qualified statement' (or vice versa) is commonly tested

4. SBA Set: Questions with keywords

- For SBA Sets, you'll come across some questions that contain a keyword - this can be used to quickly locate the relevant parts of the passage.

- If there is a keyword in the question (for an SBA Set), you probably won't need to skim for keywords in each of the statements. The keywords in the question itself should direct you to the right place in the passage.

Important Advice

- To save time, if after skimming the passage you see a change or addition of a qualifier/absolute, discard true and decide between 'False and Can't tell'.
- Numbers crop up frequently in VR, and normally you'll need to do a bit of simple math in order to attain a match between the statement and passage.

5. Questions that have a reversal

- These questions usually contain a word which results in a reversal in the way you answer it - put simply, you must do the opposite of what you're normally used to doing.

Commonly asked questions include:

- Which of the following CANNOT be true?
- Which of the following is UNLIKELY to be true?
- Make sure you adjust just the way you approach each statement - look for a false statement:

Cannot be true	Unlikely to be true/Least likely to be true
FALSE = Correct Answer	FALSE/CAN'T TELL = Correct Answer
TRUE/CAN'T TELL = Incorrect Answer	TRUE = Incorrect Answer

6. Question with no keywords

- If the question doesn't contain any keywords, you will need to skim for keywords from each statement.
- These types of questions will take longer (you may have to skim for keywords for each statement) and can be quite time-consuming. When you're running out of time, prioritise 'keyword questions' and consider skipping these questions.

Practice Questions

And here's a bucket load of practice questions to start with! It can be a bit tricky to get the method working at first - so we've tried to leave you lots of space to make notes. Loads of our students write directly in the book so that everything's in one place - see if it helps!

There are 11 questions here for you to have a go at - so if you do want to come back and do them as a practice test at some point, you can always write your notes and answers on a sheet of paper 😊

Set 1

Many people use the terms Internet and World Wide Web, or just the Web, interchangeably, but the two terms are not synonymous. The World Wide Web is a global set of documents, images and other resources, logically interrelated by hyperlinks and referenced with Uniform Resource Identifiers (URIs). URIs symbolically identify services, servers and other databases, and the documents and resources that they can provide. Hypertext Transfer Protocol (HTTP) is the main access protocol of the World Wide Web, but it is only one of the hundreds of communication protocols used on the Internet. Web services also use HTTP to allow software systems to communicate in order to share and exchange business logic and data.

World Wide Web browser software such as Microsoft's Internet Explorer, Mozilla Firefox, Opera, Apple's Safari and Google Chrome, lets users navigate from one web page to another via hyperlinks embedded in the documents. These documents may also contain any combination of computer data, including graphics, sounds, text, video, multimedia and interactive content that runs while the user is interacting with the page. Client-side software can include animations, games, office applications and scientific demonstrations. Through keyword-driven Internet research using search engines like Yahoo! and Google, users worldwide have easy, instant access to a vast and diverse amount of online information. Compared to printed media, books, encyclopedias and traditional libraries, the World Wide Web has enabled the decentralization of information on a large scale.

The Web has also enabled individuals and organizations to publish ideas and information to a potentially large audience online at greatly reduced expense and time delay. Publishing a web page, a blog, or building a website involves little initial cost and many cost-free services are available. However, publishing and maintaining large, professional web sites with attractive, diverse and up-to-date information is still a difficult and expensive proposition.

1. People can navigate the World Wide Web using all browser software.

A. True

B. False

C. Can't Tell

2. Some money is always required to build a website.

A. True

B. False

C. Can't Tell

3. The World Wide Web is often accessed via HTTP.

A. True

B. False

C. Can't Tell

4. More people use the World Wide Web in comparison to printed media and books.

A. True

B. False

C. Can't Tell

Set 2

In music, the pitch of musical sounds was perceived long before the physical basis for pitch was understood. One of the great musical (and psychological) discoveries is that for periodic musical sounds, such as those produced by the organ, strings, winds, and the human voice, pitch is tied unalterably to the periodicity or frequency with which the waveform of the sound repeats.

Periodic musical sounds are made up of many harmonically related frequency components, or partials, of frequencies fo, 2fo, 3fo, 4fo, and so forth. Such sounds have many perceived qualities besides pitch. One of these other qualities is shrillness, or brightness. A sound with intense high-low-frequency partials is bright, or shrill. A sound in which low-frequency partials predominate is not bright, but dull.

When you listen to periodic musical sounds on a hi-fi system, you can change the brightness by turning the tone control. But this doesn't change the pitch. The brightness depends on the relative intensities of partials of various frequencies. Turning the tone control can change the relations of the partials, but won't change the periodicity of the sound, which is the same as the fundamental, the frequency of the first partial, fo.

Sounds that are not periodic musical sounds are not as clear and distinguishable in pitch and
30 brightness, but some of them can be granted pitch by a sort of musical courtesy. Among these are sine waves (pure tones), the tones of bells, the clucking sound that we can make with the tongue and the roof of the mouth, the somewhat related sound of the Jew's harp, and the sound of a band of noise.

Sine waves are peculiar in that they consist of a single harmonic partial. The sense of pitch that they give is not as certain as that of other periodic sounds; it can differ a little with intensity, and between the two ears. For other periodic sounds, the sense of the octave is very strong, for the partials of a sound a' (that is, an octave above a) are all present in sound a. The sense of the octave is not strong with sine waves. Furthermore, because sine waves contain only one frequency component, their brightness is tied inextricably to their pitch.

1. The periodicity of a musical sound is built from harmonically related frequency components.
A. True
B. False
C. Can't Tell

2. Sine waves consist of several harmonic frequencies.
A. True
B. False
C. Can't Tell

3. Turning the tone control won't change the frequency of the first partial.
A. True
B. False
C. Can't Tell

4. Increasing the amplitude of a wave will increase the volume of a musical sound.
A. True
B. False
C. Can't Tell

Set 3

To the surprise of scientists, giant endangered fish with saw-like snouts in Florida are experiencing virgin births, reproducing without sex. This is the first solid evidence of such asexual reproduction in the wild for any animal with a backbone.

Asexual reproduction is often seen among invertebrates – that is, animals without backbones. It happens rarely in vertebrates, but instances are increasingly being discovered. For example, the Komodo dragon, the world's largest living lizard, has given birth via parthenogenesis, in which an unfertilized egg develops to maturity. Such virgin births have also been seen in sharks, in birds such as chickens and turkeys, and in snakes such as pit vipers and boa constrictors. Such virgin-born offspring are known as parthenogens.

Until now, evidence of parthenogenesis in vertebrates came nearly entirely from captive animals, usually surprising their keepers by giving birth despite the fact that they had not had any mates. Scientists had recently found two female snakes in the wild that were each pregnant with progeny that developed via parthenogenesis, but it was not known if these parthenogens would have survived. As such, it remained uncertain whether virgin births happened to any significant extent in nature.

Small tooth sawfish are one of five species of sawfish, a group of large rays known for long, tooth-studded snouts that the animals use to subdue small fish. Small tooth sawfish are mainly found nowadays in a handful of locations in southwest Florida. Recent DNA fingerprinting of the sawfish was conducted in this area in order to see if relatives were often reproducing with relatives due to their small population size. Andrew Fields and colleagues found that DNA fingerprints revealed female sawfish to be sometimes reproducing without mating.

1. Sawfish are the only type of fish with tooth-studded snouts.

A. True

B. False

C. Can't Tell

2. Parthenogenesis is more commonly observed in animals lacking a backbone.

A. True

B. False

C. Can't Tell

3. Andrew Fields is a leading marine biologist.

A. True

B. False

C. Can't Tell

4. Evidence of parthenogenesis among wild snakes provides convincing evidence that virgin births often occur in the wild.

A. True

B. False

C. Can't Tell

Set 4

The Sholes and Glidden typewriter was the first commercially successful typewriter. Principally designed by the American inventor Christopher Latham Sholes, it was developed with the assistance of fellow printer Samuel W. Soule and amateur mechanic Carlos S. Glidden. Development began in 1867, but Soule left the enterprise shortly thereafter, replaced by James Densmore, who provided financial backing and the driving force behind the machine's continued development. After several short-lived attempts to manufacture the device, the machine was acquired by E. Remington and Sons in early 1873. An arms manufacturer seeking to diversify, Remington further refined the typewriter before finally placing it on the market on July 1, 1874.

During its development, the typewriter evolved from a crude curiosity into a practical device, the basic form of which became the industry standard. The machine incorporated elements, which became fundamental to typewriter design, including a cylindrical platen and a four-rowed QWERTY keyboard. Several design deficiencies remained, however. The Sholes and Glidden could print only upper-case letters—an issue remedied in its successor, the Remington No. 2— and was a "blind writer", meaning the typist could not see what was being written as it was entered.

Initially, the typewriter received an unenthusiastic reception from the public. Lack of an established market, high cost, and the need for trained operators slowed its adoption. Additionally, recipients of typewritten messages found the mechanical, all upper-case writing to be impersonal and even insulting. The new communication technologies and expanding businesses of the late 19th century, however, had created a need for expedient, legible correspondence, and so the Sholes and Glidden and its contemporaries soon became common office fixtures. The typewriter is credited with assisting the entrance of women into the clerical workplace, as many were hired to operate the new devices.

1. Typewriter sales began in 1867.

A. True

B. False

C. Can't Tell

2. When the typewriter was initially introduced, more people still preferred to alternative mediums of writing.

A. True

B. False

C. Can't Tell

3. Remington addressed some of the design faults in the original typewriter.

A. True

B. False

C. Can't Tell

4. After the rise of typewriters as office fixtures, the operation of typewriters in the workplace was largely by women.

A. True

B. False

C. Can't Tell

The potential application of xenografting arises because in recent years there has been an increase in the number of heart transplantations to the point that demand significantly exceeds any reasonable expectation of the routine "supply" of suitable hearts from cadavers. By definition, patients who would benefit from heart transplantation are critically ill. Hence the limitation in supply inevitably means than some people will die before a suitable organ becomes available. This suggests an ethical motive for this research.

Genetic manipulation has become involved as a possible way of preventing the hyperacute response whereby human antibodies act rapidly to reject the transplanted tissue as though responding to an infection. Current research is attempting to transfer the gene which directs the production of regulatory factors for human "complement" into pigs, so that the heart is no longer recognized as foreign.

Conventional drug therapy is, however, still required to minimize rejection by response to the histocompatibility antigens, which react to the different tissue surface chemicals of an organ transplanted even within the same species. The actual technique being used involves a single gene (it is presumed without a regulator). There appear to be several groups of people working on the technique and different groups appear to have chosen different genes to work with. A group from Cambridge was still some way from applying the technology to human recipients. In early 1995, they were only at the stage of producing homozygous lines of transgenic pigs. Other groups have gone further in the genetic engineering aspects, but none are at a clinical trial stage.

1. The increase in the number of heart transplantations is due to an increasing number of people adopting unhealthy lifestyles.
A. True
B. False
C. Can't Tell

2. A problem in heart transplantation is the host antibody response to the transplanted tissue.
A. True
B. False
C. Can't Tell

3. Gene manipulation can have an effect on histocompatibility antigen incompatibility.
A. True
B. False
C. Can't Tell

4. Drug therapy is currently used to reduce rejection of a transplanted heart by the host.
A. True
B. False
C. Can't Tell

In December world leaders gathered in Kyoto, Japan, to grapple with the growing threat of global warming caused by the burning of fossil fuels. To combat the surge in greenhouse gases, chiefly carbon dioxide researchers and policymakers have called for energy conservation, taxes on carbon emissions and the swift development of renewable energy sources, such as wind and solar power. Still, with nuclear energy out of favour and no easy replacement for fossil fuels on the horizon, the rise in atmospheric carbon dioxide might appear unstoppable. But a growing number of scientists are pointing out that another means of combating greenhouse warming may be at hand, one that deals with the problem rather directly: put the carbon back where it came from, into the earth.

The idea of somehow "sequestering" carbon is not new. One method is simply to grow more trees, which take carbon from the atmosphere and convert it to woody matter. Although the extent of planting would have to be enormous, William R. Moomaw, a physical chemist at Tufts University, estimates that 10 to 15 percent of the carbon dioxide problem could be solved in this way.

Howard J. Herzog of the Massachusetts Institute of Technology proposes pumping carbon dioxide into the deep ocean. Although the tactic might be viewed as exchanging one form of pollution for another, there are good reasons to consider making the trade. The ocean contains at least three times more carbon than the atmosphere does, so adding the carbon dioxide from the burning of fossil fuels to the sea would have a proportionally smaller effect. Advocates of this fix also point out that much of the carbon dioxide now released finds its way into the ocean anyway, disturbing the chemistry of the surface waters.

Rather than sequestering carbon dioxide in the sea, other researchers argue the carbon should be returned to the ground. Many natural gas deposits already contain huge quantities of carbon dioxide. So, it is unlikely that pumping in more would harm the subterranean environment. And petroleum engineers are already well versed in the mechanics of this operation. For years oil companies have taken carbon dioxide from underground deposits and injected it into deep-seated formations to aid in flushing oil from dwindling reservoirs.

1. Carbon dioxide is a significant contributor to the surge in greenhouse gases.

A. True

B. False

C. Can't Tell

2. By the time it takes to grow enough trees, the situation could reach an irreparable stage.

A. True

B. False

C. Can't Tell

3. The ocean is more likely to be able to contain more carbon dioxide than the natural gas deposits underground.

A. True

B. False

C. Can't Tell

4. Carbon dioxide is often used to remove any remaining oil underground.

A. True

B. False

C. Can't Tell

Set 7

The study of psychology in a philosophical context dates back to the ancient civilizations of Egypt, Greece, China, India, and Persia. Historians note that Greek philosophers, including Thales, Plato, and Aristotle, covered the workings of the mind in their writings. As early as the 4th century BC, Greek physician Hippocrates theorized that mental disorders were of a physical, rather than divine, nature.

German physician Wilhelm Wundt is credited with introducing psychological discovery into an experimental setting. Known as the "father of experimental psychology", he founded the first psychological laboratory, at Leipzig University, in 1879 - Wundt, focusing on breaking down mental processes into the most basic components, was motivated in part by an analogy to recent advances in chemistry, and its successful investigation of the elements and structure of material.

From the 1890s until his death in 1939, the Austrian physician Sigmund Freud developed psychoanalysis, which comprised a method of investigating the mind and interpreting experience; a systematized set of theories about human behaviour; and a form of psychotherapy thought to treat psychological or emotional distress, especially unconscious conflict. Contrast this with the newer, more widely used psychotherapies - such as Cognitive Behavioural Therapy, Cognitive Analytical Therapy and Interpersonal Psychotherapy, requiring the subject to see their therapist once a week.

In the United States, behaviourism became the dominant school of thought during the 1950s: a discipline that was established in the early 20th century by John Watson. It posited that behavioural tendencies are determined by immediate associations between various environmental stimuli and the degree of pleasure or pain that follows. Behavioural patterns, then, were understood to involve organisms' conditioned responses to the stimuli in their environment.

1. Which of the following statements is least likely to be true?

A. Hippocrates proposed that disorders of the mind had a physical origin.

B. Psychoanalysis is a dated form of psychotherapy.

C. Watson is credited with the establishment of behaviourism.

D. Psychology was first studied in Ancient Greece.

2. Which of the following statements is true?

A. Behavioural tendencies depend upon the generation of pleasant or painful emotions in response to internal stimuli.

B. Scientific progress in the 19th century played a role in inspiring Wundt to bring the study of Psychology into the experimental realm.

C. Behaviourism was established towards the end of the 20th century.

D. Aristotle played a major role in the foundations underlying psychology.

3. Which of the following statements can be inferred from the passage?

A. Behaviourist theories play a prominent role in psychology today.

B. A behaviourist would argue that our behavioural patterns are guided by rewarding and aversive stimuli.

C. Behaviourist theories were influenced by Freud's experimental work during the early 20th century.

D. A conditioned response to external stimuli is sufficient to produce behavioural patterns.

4. Which of the following statements is false?

A. Psychoanalysis used in psychotherapy has been proposed to be able to resolve unconscious conflict.

B. Therapists offering Cognitive Analytical Therapy require subjects to undergo therapy once a month.

C. Wundt established the first psychological laboratory.

D. Sigmund Freud died in 1939.

Set 8

Childhood developmental refers to biological, psychological and emotional changes that occur following birth, right the way through to adolescence. It is a continuous process with a predictable sequence. Every child develops in their own unique way, and under the influence of genetic and environmental factors. Genetically-controlled processes are known as 'maturation' whilst the child 'learns' from environmental factors. Usually, there is a strong interaction between the two.

Typically, the first learnt social interaction is the smile, which starts at about 6 weeks of age. In the first few months, newborns do not seem to experience fear, and only experience happiness, sadness, and anger. Around the age of about 10 months, there is a fairly rapid development, and they can be fearful of perceived threats, prefer familiar people and situations, and exhibit separation anxiety.

The understanding of speech develops gradually from about 6 months. Expressive language – the ability to produce words – begins around 12 months and accelerates rapidly at 18 months. By 2 years, children produce three or four worded sentences, and at 3 years can produce complex sentences. By 5 years, most are able to use language in similar ways to an adult.

Delays in language development are more common in boys than girls. Simple delays are usually temporary and resolve on their own. Occasionally delays can be due to more serious conditions such as auditory processing disorders or autism. Hearing impairment is one of the most common causes of language delay, although sign language can often develop at the same pace as language in children that can hear.

1. According to the passage, which of the following statements best apply to a child's development?
A. From birth, there are intervals, or pauses, in a child's development.
B. Psychological development is not dependent on the mother.
C. Genetic maturation and environmental factors both have an influence on the development of children.
D. Psychological development is linked inherently with emotional changes.

2. Which of the following is a common cause of language delay, according to the passage?
A. Cerebral infarction
B. Autism
C. Auditory processing disorders
D. Hearing impairment

3. According to the passage, which of the following is least likely to be true?
A. During development, a child's maturation is due to genetically controlled processes.
B. Newborns do not appear to have a fear response.
C. No children under the age of 12 months have the ability to use expressive language.
D. Newborns are not able to smile in a social context until around 6 weeks of age.

4. Which of the following, regarding the understanding of speech, is most likely to be correct, according to the passage?
A. The use of expressive language begins to increase quickly around 15 month's age.
B. A child can produce longer, more difficult, sentences around 3 years of age.
C. A child is unable to produce three worded sentences at 2 years of age
D. It would take at least 6 years for most children to be able to produce any language similar to that of an adult.

The Cetacean suborder Mysticeti includes the blue, humpback, bowhead and minke whales. These whales are filter feeders, eating small organisms which are removed from seawater by a comb-like structure inside the mouth known as a baleen. Their forelimbs are fins and their nasal openings form their blowhole. Like all mammals, whales breathe air, are warm blooded, produce milk for their young and have body hair.

The blue whale is the largest animal known to have existed and can grow to 30m in length and weigh 180 tonnes. There are at least 3 different subspecies found in all the different oceans of the world. They feed almost exclusively on zooplankton and an adult blue whale can eat up to 40 million krill, or 3600 Kg in a day.

They hunt krill at depths of about 100m during the day and at the surface at night. Hunting dives can last for up to 30 minutes at a time. Blue whales themselves are so large they have virtually no natural predators, although up to a quarter of blue whales have scars from orca (killer whale) attacks.

A whale's gestation period is 12 months and females give birth every two to three years to a calf that can weigh 3 tonnes. Sexual maturity is reached at about 7 years and total lifespan could be over 100 years, although no studies have been lengthy enough to ascertain this for certain.

In 2002, there were an estimated 8000 blue whales worldwide. Their numbers were decimated by commercial whaling in the 19th and early 20th centuries, reducing the population from an approximate 800,000 worldwide. Since the introduction of the whaling ban, best estimates show an increase of 7.3 % per year but numbers remain at under 1% of what they were pre-whaling.

1. The passage supports which of the following conclusions?
A. Krill descend during the day and come to the surface at night.
B. The blue whale is the largest animal that has ever existed.
C. Bowhead whale population drastically decreased due to commercial whaling in the 19th century.
D. Blue whales sometimes feed on other things aside from Zooplankton.

2. Using information from the passage, we can infer that:
A. The whaling ban has had little effect on the blue whale population.
B. Krill are a type of Zooplankton.
C. Female blue whales give birth at least once a month.
D. Some blue whales are killed by sharks every year.

3. Which of the following statements about mammals are false?
A. Minke whales are a type of mammal.
B. All whales are warm-blooded.
C. Like monkeys, whales have body hair.
D. Some types of mammal do not produce milk for their young.

4. Referring to the passage, all of these statements are true, except:
A. Due to their size, blue whales have few natural predators.
B. Whales can reproduce 9 years from birth after having reached sexual maturity.
C. The population of all the different types of whales in the suborder Mysticeti was reduced by whaling.
D. Bowhead whales could potentially live more than 100 years.

Set 10

Alcoholism is a broad term for any drinking of alcohol that results in a wide range of possible problems. In a medical context, alcoholism is said to exist when two or more of the following is present: a person drinks large amounts over a long time period, has difficulty cutting down, acquiring and drinking alcohol takes up a great deal of time, alcohol is strongly desired, usage results in not fulfilling responsibilities, usage results in social problems and/or health problems, withdrawal occurs when stopping, and tolerance has occurred to use.

Both environmental factors and genetics are involved in causing alcoholism with about half the risk attributed to each. A person with a parent or sibling who is alcoholic are three to four times more likely to become alcoholic themselves. Environmental factors include social, cultural, and behavioural influences. High stress levels, anxiety, as well as inexpensive easily accessible alcohol, increases risk. People dependent on alcohol typically continue to drink partly to prevent or improve symptoms of withdrawal.

Prevention of alcoholism is possible by regulating and limiting the sale of alcohol, taxing alcohol to increase its cost, and providing inexpensive treatment. Treatment may take several steps. Because of the severe medical problems that can occur during withdrawal, alcohol detoxification should be carefully controlled. After detoxification, support such as group therapy or self-help groups are used to help keep a person from returning to drinking.

Alcohol accounts for 6% of all hospital admissions in the UK. In 2012, there were roughly 8,000 alcohol-related deaths in the UK. Moreover, males accounted for approximately 70% of all alcohol-related deaths in the UK in 2012. Interestingly, men and women prisoners who reported drinking daily drank an average of 20 units a day. Statistics show that victims believed offenders to be under the influence of alcohol in around 900,000 offenses, which is roughly half of all reported violent incidents in a year.

1. Using information in the passage, the writer would probably most agree with which one of the following?
A. Alcohol accounts for approximately 400,000 hospital admissions in the UK.
B. Both male and female prisoners on average report drinking 200 units a month.
C. Males accounted for roughly 5,600 alcohol-related deaths in the UK in 2012.
D. There are around 1.5 million violent incidents a year.

2. Which of the following statements is false?
A. Limiting access to alcohol can play a part in reducing alcoholism.
B. The alleviation of withdrawal symptoms is not common reason for continuing drinking habits amongst alcoholics.
C. The increasing numbers of young offenders may be a result of corresponding increases in alcohol consumption amongst young people.
D. Treatment for alcoholics is not always a simple, single-step process.

3. According to the passage, the author would LEAST likely agree with which one of the following?
A. A person with trouble reducing alcohol consumption and who cannot fulfil day-to-day responsibilities due to such usage can be termed alcoholic.
B. Many of the factors leading to and causing alcoholism are out of a person's control.
C. Rapid, uncontrolled detoxification in alcoholics can lead to serious health complications.
D. Group or self-help therapy is necessary for preventing a return to alcohol dependency.

4. From the passage, which of the following is true?
A. Increased pricing of alcohol will not act as a deterrent for alcoholics.
B. The risk of alcoholism can be 400% higher for a person with an alcoholic sibling.
C. Stress and anxiety play little part as factors leading to alcoholism.
D. There are more young people than adults committing alcohol-related crimes.

Scientists have known for many years that not all the charged particles in interplanetary space come from the sun. Some of the other particles are atoms stripped of their electrons and accelerated elsewhere in the galaxy to nearly the speed of light. Earthbound researchers, who have long been able to measure the more energetic fraction of these particles as they bombard the atmosphere, named the high-speed intruders cosmic rays. The earliest spacecraft measurements of cosmic rays obtained nearly four decades ago, showed that rays with lower energies than those recorded near the surface of Earth also exist in abundance. Scientists had discovered that the solar system was, in fact, awash in a variety of particles coming, it seemed, from all over the galaxy.

Researchers soon realized that the outflow of solar wind must prevent some galactic cosmic rays from approaching the sun. So only a portion of them penetrates to the inner heliosphere, where, like salmon swimming upstream to spawn, they must overcome increasingly severe obstacles. What exactly are the barriers in "empty" space? The low densities of material indeed ensure that cosmic rays and solar-wind particles do not actually collide. After the solar wind leaves the vicinity of the sun, however, it carries part of the solar magnetic field along with it. So incoming rays are subject to the forces that magnetic fields exert on electrically charged particles in motion. Such forces cause cosmic rays to wrap around the magnetic field lines as they simultaneously drift along the field direction. The circling rays can also encounter magnetic waves, which propagate along the magnetic-field lines in a manner resembling the fluttering of a flag. These waves cause the direction of the magnetic field to shift abruptly, thereby impeding the flow of charged particles. In effect, a cosmic ray headed toward the sun is like a swimmer trying to enter the ocean in the presence of strong surf.

Before the Ulysses mission, astronomers speculated that cosmic rays traveling inward over the poles of the sun might penetrate the heliosphere more easily than those that followed more equatorial routes. There were two principal reasons for this surmise. First, because charged particles follow a helical path along magnetic field lines, they had expected the shorter, straighter lines of force connecting with the poles to be excellent conduits into the inner heliosphere. Second, some researchers believed waves and other disturbing changes in field direction would be minimal, because the solar wind from coronal holes flows comparatively smoothly.

1. According to the passage, which of the following is most likely to be true?
A. All charged particles in interplanetary space originate from the sun.
B. Cosmic rays are slow moving particles that enter the atmosphere.
C. Removing electrons from an atom can be achieved by accelerating it to near the speed of light.
D. The cosmic rays recorded near the surface of the earth tend to be high energy particles.

2. Which of the following is the best reason cosmic rays are prevented from fully penetrating the sun, according to the passage?
A. There is a strong 'surf' of UV rays, from the solar wind, that diverts incoming rays.
B. Solar wind outflow directly acts as an obstacle to cosmic rays.
C. A magnetic field carried by solar wind outflow which distorts the path of incoming rays.
D. An abundance of low density material in 'empty space'.

3. Which of the following would the author most agree with?
A. It is equally difficult for cosmic rays to penetrate the heliosphere.
B. Coronal holes can be found over the poles of the sun.
C. Charged particles don't follow a distinct path along magnetic field lines.
D. The lines of force connecting with the poles of the sun are weak channels for cosmic rays to penetrate the sun.

4. According to the passage, which of the following is most likely to be true?
A. The heliosphere surrounds the sun.
B. Cosmic rays can only be measured by people in spacecraft.
C. Solar wind is caused by a similar mechanism controlling wind on Earth.
D. Most cosmic rays penetrate the inner heliosphere.

Solutions

<u>True/False Sets Initial Example</u>

1. True

The London Underground is the oldest underground system in the world.

Effective Keywords: Oldest, World, London Underground

Skimming for 'oldest', we are told in the first paragraph that "It is the world's oldest and longest underground system". Some of you may know the answer to this from your own general knowledge - but be very careful, ensure it's referenced in the passage. If it were not referenced in the passage, even if you know that it is the oldest, the answer would be 'Cant Tell'.

2.False

It is estimated that the total passenger count on the Underground in a year will reach one billion, for the first time, in 2020.

Effective Keywords: 2020, One Billion

If we skim for '2020' we can't find it anywhere in the passage, whereas 'one billion ' appears near the end of the second paragraph, where we are told that one billion passengers were recorded in 2007. It is therefore false to say that it will happen for the first time in 2020.

3 Can't Tell

There are over 100 ventilation shafts along the Underground network.

Effective Keywords: 100, Ventilation Shafts

Again, if we skim for '100', we can't find anything in the passage. We are told in the final paragraph that ventilation shafts exist - but there is no reference to how many there are.

4. True

A greater proportion of the London Underground network is above ground than below ground.

Effective Keywords: Above/Below Ground

The keyword 'above ground' appears near the middle of the first paragraph where we are told that 55% of the network is above ground. Therefore, this statement is true.

SBA Sets Initial Example

1. Shoots

Which of the following is listed by the passage as being eaten by the Western gorilla but not by the Eastern gorilla?

Effective keywords: Eaten, Western Gorilla, Eastern Gorilla

Upon assessing this SBA question, we can see straight away that it provides an array of useful keywords and is looking for a comparison to be made. The two types of Gorilla, 'Western' and 'Eastern' are good words to skim for, and you should also keep in mind the main point of the statement, that is what these gorillas 'eat'. Skimming for these words leads us to the first passage, but on checking the context of the sentence containing these words, we find no mention of 'eating' or anything synonymous to it. On further skimming, we're led to the second paragraph, where we are told that Western gorillas eat leaves, stems, pith and shoots and a small amount of fruit. We are then told that the Eastern gorilla eats leaves, pith, termites, ants, aquatic herbs and large amounts of fruit. It is clear that shoots are the only food that the Western gorilla eats that the Eastern gorilla does not. This question demonstrates how you can save time by quickly taking advantage of effective keyword selection from the question itself and skimming the passage for relevant information.

2. Silverback gorillas typically weigh twice as much as female gorillas.

According to the passage, which of the following is most likely to be false?

Remember, for this question, we are looking for something that is likely to be False. We can therefore only discard statements that we know are true. The answer doesn't necessarily have to be false- a statement that is 'can't tell' is more likely false than a statement that is 'true'. This is a classic way in which the UKCAT VR section can confuse students.

> A: The gorilla can be broken down to distinct species which can be further broken down into sub-species.

Effective Keywords: Species, Sub-species

Evaluating this statement, the important keywords relate to the 'species' of gorilla, and its subdivision. Skimming for these words, we're led to the first paragraph, where we are told that, "The eponymous genus Gorilla is divided into two species, the Eastern gorilla and the Western gorilla, and either four or five subspecies". This statement is therefore true, and it's a simple case of the statement rewording information from the passage. Remember to discard because we're looking for a statement that is False.

> B: Silverback gorillas have been known to sacrifice themselves to protect their troop.

Effective Keywords: Silverback, Sacrifice, Protect

The most useful and unique keyword in this statement is firstly the 'Silverback' gorilla, and then the idea of its willingness for 'sacrifice' in order to 'protect'. Keep all these words in mind and look for synonyms or similar ideas in the passage as you skim. Indeed, we're led to the third paragraph, which tells us that silverbacks will protect the group "even at the cost of his own life". Again, this is another case of the statement rewording the passage, making it quite clearly true. Discard and continue looking for the false statement.

C: Gorillas do not typically need to drink water.

Effective Keywords: Water, Drink

Clearly, the statement boils down to gorillas 'drinking water', and so these keywords should promise to be the most high-yield. Skimming the passage, we're told in the second paragraph that gorillas rarely drink water because they can obtain their daily requirements through eating "succulent vegetation". The statement and passage clearly agree with each other, and it's another simple case of rewording. This statement is therefore true, and we can immediately select option d) as the answer because we know that all statements so far have been true. You must be able to ruthlessly and confidently decide on answers in the exam to save time - don't even try to work out the last statement and move on to the next question (although the answer is provided).

D: Silverback gorillas typically weigh twice as much as female gorillas.

Effective Keywords: Silverback, Female, Weight

Firstly, the best keywords here are most likely 'Silverback', alongside its comparison to 'female' gorillas in terms of 'weight'. Skimming the passage, there is actually no reference to the weight of the gorillas at all: the statement makes a comparison that is not supported by the passage, and is therefore most likely to be false.

3. Video footage showing a silverback 'bluff charging' an attacking leopard.

Which of the following considerations is not listed by the passage as supporting the theory that the leopard preys on the gorilla?

Effective Keywords: Leopard, Preys, Gorilla

You have to be careful here, this question is looking for a statement that is not listed by the passage as supporting the theory laid out in the question. This means that it must be either a statement that states information beyond the scope of the passage, a false statement that directly contradicts the passage or a true statement that does not support this theory.

You also have valuable keywords in the question itself, namely the 'leopard preying' on the 'gorilla'. Skimming for this, we can quickly find 'predator' in the final paragraph, along with 'leopard' and 'gorilla'. On comparison with each of the statements, it's clear that a), b) and c) are all consistent with the paragraph and do provide support for the predatory nature of leopards against gorillas. d) therefore must be the correct answer - certainly references are made to bluff charging as a defensive mechanism, but there is no reference to video footage capturing said charge, thus this is not 'listed in the passage as supporting the theory that the leopard preys on the gorilla'.

4. The gorilla and the human share upwards of 95% of their DNA.

According to the passage, which of the following statements is true?

A: The gorilla and the human share upwards of 95% of their DNA.

Effective Keywords: 95%, DNA, (Gorilla), (Human)

Upon evaluating the statement, we can see straightaway that there are fantastic keywords to skim for, specifically the percentage '95%' and the abbreviation 'DNA'. Also keep in mind what you're actually comparing: 'humans' and 'gorillas'. Skimming for these high-yield keywords, we find these words in the first paragraph tells us that "The DNA of gorillas is highly similar to that of humans, from 95-99% depending on what is counted". Thus, the statement has simply reworded the passage, and thus is true. This is the answer to this question - ensure you don't waste time evaluating the other three options: discard, and move on to the next set in order to save as much time as possible!

> B: Western gorillas must travel further each day to scavenge for food than the Eastern gorilla.

This is false because it directly contradicts the passage - we are told in the second paragraph that it is the Eastern gorilla that must travel far and wide, and not the Western gorilla.

> C: The gorilla is the closest living relative to humans.

Again, this is contradicts the passage and is therefore false. We are told in the first paragraph that both the chimpanzee and the bonobo are closer living relatives to humans than the gorilla.

> D: Gorillas sleep in nests in the trees.

There is no reference within the passage to where gorillas sleep.

1. Can't tell

'People can navigate the World Wide Web using all browser software.'

Keywords: Browser Software

The relevant information can be found at the beginning of the second paragraph. The passage states that indeed 'browser software... lets users navigate from one web page to another via hyperlinks', however we cannot extrapolate to all browsers. Note the absolute language, and because the information needed to answer this question is beyond the passage, the answer is can't tell.

2. False

'Some money is always required to build a website.'

Keywords: Website, (Money)

Skimming for 'website', which forms an important part of the statement, leads us to the last paragraph. Note the absolute language in this statement: - 'always' - and so it is important to be cautious. Indeed, the passage directly contradicts the statement, with 'many cost-free services' available for 'building a website'. Thus, the answer is false.

3. True

'The World Wide Web is often accessed via HTTP.'

Keywords to skim for: HTTP, (World Wide Web)

You'll find the relevant section towards the end of the first paragraph - it is better to skim for HTTP, because it's an abbreviation (making it stick out) and also as World Wide Web is highly prevalent throughout the passage. Based on the language used and the context, it's in agreement. Note the usage of the word 'often' in the statement; this does not imply usage is more than 50%, it merely suggests it is frequently used. The passage states HTTP is the 'main' access protocol, which assures the validity of the statement. If another word such as 'usually' or 'most often' is used instead - we cannot be as sure based on the information in the passage. Thus, the answer is true.

4. Can't tell

'More people use the World Wide Web in comparison to printed media and books.'

Keywords: Books, Printed Media

Skimming for 'books' leads us to the end of the second paragraph: but the relevant sentence talks about how the WWW enabled the redistribution of information in comparison to 'printed media' and 'books. This does not relate to the question statement, and whether more people use the WWW than printed media and books require information that is beyond the passage: thus, the safest answer is can't tell.

1. True

'The periodicity of a musical sound is built from harmonically related frequency components. '

Keywords: Periodicity, Harmonically related frequency

You'll find the relevant section around the middle of the first paragraph. The passage states 'periodic musical sounds are made up of harmonically related frequency components'; this is a direct agreement.

2. False

'Sine waves consist of several harmonic frequencies.'

Keywords: Sine waves, (Harmonic frequencies)

You'll find the relevant section around the middle of the last paragraph (the keyword 'Sine' appears twice). The passage states: 'Sine waves... consist of a single harmonic partial'; this contradicts the statement which suggested there were 'several' harmonic frequencies. Moreover, it's the harmonic partial, which is relevant, not the frequency.

3. True

'Turning the tone control won't change the frequency of the first partial.'

Keywords: Tone control, (First partial)

You'll find the relevant section at the end of the second paragraph. Again, 'tone control' is mentioned several times, but skimming should have led you to the relevant part. The passage states: 'Turning the tone control...won't change the periodicity of the sound, which is the same as the fundamental, the frequency of the first partial'; this is in direct agreement.

4. Can't tell

'Increasing the amplitude of a wave will increase the volume of a musical sound.'

Keywords: Amplitude, Wave, Volume

None of these keywords appear in the passage. Even without reading the whole passage, we can assume the answer is 'Can't tell'. It is tempting to overthink and rationalize the statement, but if you read initially and it is not fitting it then do not waste time.

1. Can't tell

'Sawfish are the only type of fish with tooth-studded snouts.'

Keywords: Sawfish, Tooth-studded snouts

Skimming for either 'sawfish' or 'snouts' leads us to first sentence of the final paragraph. Although we are told that sawfish are known for 'long tooth-studded snouts', this does not necessarily mean no other types of fish have tooth studded snouts. Beware of the absolute language used: 'only'. Thus, we require further information, and the answer is can't tell.

2. True

'Parthenogenesis is more commonly observed in animals lacking a backbone.'

Keywords: Parthenogenesis, backbone

The keyword 'parthenogenesis' is a striking one, and leads us to the second paragraph, which explains it to effectively means the development of virgin-born offspring as a result of asexual reproduction. The first sentence of that paragraph indicates that this process is 'often' seen among invertebrates - but crucially, it happens 'rarely' in vertebrates. Even though discovered instances are increasing among vertebrates, the passage makes it clear that Parthenogenesis is more commonly observed in animals lacking a backbone, and thus the passage agrees with the statement: the answer is true.

3. Can't tell

'Andrew Fields is a leading marine biologist.'

Keywords: Andrew Fields

Names are easy to scan for and skimming 'Andrew Fields' immediately leads us to the last sentence of the last paragraph. Based on the context of the paragraph, it is reasonable to think that Andrew Fields is a marine biologist, however whether he is a 'leading' marine biologist is another matter. Indeed, we do not know whether he is a 'leading' marine biologist or not based on the information in the passage, and so the safest bet is to put 'can't tell'.

3. False

'Evidence of parthenogenesis among wild snakes provides convincing evidence that virgin births often

occur in the wild.'

Keywords: Snakes

The keyword in this statement is 'snakes' because it plays an important, unique role. Skimming for it leads us to the third paragraph, and indeed there is evidence that 'progeny' had development via parthenogenesis. However, the next sentence importantly states that whether this process happens to 'any significant extent' in the wild remains uncertain, which is a direct contradiction to the question statement. Thus, the answer is false.

Set 4

1. False

'Typewriter sales began in 1867.'

Keywords: 1867

The best keyword for this question is '1867', which we can easily skim for; this brings us to the middle of the first paragraph - however, this part of the passage does not give any indication of typewriter sales during this time. Instead, reading the rest of the paragraph reveals that the typewriter was placed on the market in 1874, not 1867, thus the answer is false.

2. True

'When the typewriter was initially introduced, most people still preferred alternative mediums of writing.'

Keywords: Handwrite, (Typewriter)

We can pick out two keywords here: 'typewriter' and 'handwrite'; however, 'typewriter' appears throughout the passage, making it difficult to locate the relevant context, and 'handwrite' is not mentioned in the passage. These questions that lack high-yield keywords are generally more rare, and we recommend skipping these if you're low on time: it is tempting to put 'can't tell', however the beginning of the third paragraph states that the typewriter 'received an unenthusiastic reception from the public'. We can infer from this that, at least initially, most people did not adopt the typewriter and used the only alternative medium of writing, which is by hand. Thus, the answer is true.

3. True

'Remington addressed some of the design faults in the original typewriter.'

Keywords: Remington, Design

If we were to just skim for 'Remington', we know from the first paragraph that Remington 'further refined' the typewriter, but not whether any design faults were actually fixed. Skimming for 'Remington' and 'design' together brings us to the end of the second paragraph; reading the context reveals that there were in fact 'design deficiencies' in the Scholes and Glidden typewriter, and that this remedied in the Remington No.2. Thus, this is in agreement with the question statement and the answer is true.

4. Can't tell

'After the rise of typewriters as office fixtures, the operation of typewriters in the workplace was largely by women.'

Keywords: Workplace, Women

Skimming for 'workplace' brings us to the end of the passage, which states that the typewriter 'assisted in brining women into the clerical workplace' and 'many were hired to operate' these devices. However, the question statement indicates that the majority of people operating typewriters in the office were women, which simply cannot be implied from the passage. Although it is a possibility, we need more information, so the answer is can't tell.

Set 5

1. Can't Tell

'The increase in the number of heart transplantations is due to an increasing number of people adopting unhealthy lifestyles.'

Keywords: Heart transplantation, Unhealthy lifestyle

Heart transplantation appears twice in the first paragraph. There is no suggestion or mention of people adopting unhealthy lifestyles and a link to heart transplantation. This statement is beyond the passage.

2. True

'A significant problem in heart transplantation is the host antibody response to the transplanted tissue.'

Keywords: Antibody response, (Transplant)

You'll find the relevant section at the beginning of the second paragraph. We're told 'human antibodies act rapidly to reject the transplanted tissue', so this agrees with the statement.

3. Can't Tell

'Gene manipulation can have an effect on histocompatibility antigen incompatibility.'

Keywords: Histocompatibility antigen, Gene manipulation

The keyword 'histocompatibility antigen' can be found around the middle of the last paragraph. On further skimming, we find 'genetic manipulation' mentioned at the beginning of the first paragraph. From the context of the passage, gene manipulation is referring to the antibody response, whilst the histocompatibility antigen response is a separate issue (don't over-think or bring in your own knowledge). Without further information, we can't say if gene manipulation can have an effect on histocompatibility antigens, the statement is beyond the passage.

4. True

'Drug therapy is currently used to reduce rejection of a transplanted heart by the host. '

Keywords: Drug therapy, Rejection, (Transplanted heart)

You'll find the relevant section around the middle of the last paragraph. The passage states 'conventional drug therapy... is required to minimize rejection by response to the histocompatibility antigens...' - we can assume by the context ('conventional drug therapy') that this is a therapy currently used.

<u>Set 6</u>

1. True

'Carbon dioxide is a significant contributor to the surge in greenhouse gases.'

Keywords: Carbon Dioxide, Greenhouse gases

You'll find the relevant section in the second sentence of the first paragraph. From this part of the passage, 'to combat the surge in greenhouse gases, chiefly carbon dioxide...', we can imply carbon dioxide plays a major role in the surge in greenhouse gases.

2. Can't Tell

'By the time it takes to grow enough trees, the situation could reach an irreparable stage. '

Keywords: Trees, Irreparable

The relevant section can be found near the end of the first paragraph. Although the passage states 'the extent of the planting would have to be enormous', we can't tell if the planting of trees will be too slow to counteract the dangerous surge of greenhouse gasses. The statement is beyond the passage.

3. Can't Tell

'The ocean is more likely to be able to contain more carbon dioxide than the natural gas deposits underground. '

Keywords: Ocean, Natural gas deposits

In the second paragraph, the passage states 'the ocean contains at least three times more carbon than the atmosphere does', and later on, in the final paragraph, it states 'many natural gas deposits already contain huge quantities of carbon dioxide'. Although both areas in the passage suggest a large potential store for carbon dioxide, it is beyond the passage to determine which will be able to contain more carbon dioxide.

4. True

'Carbon dioxide is often used to remove any remaining oil underground.'

Keywords: Oil, Carbon Dioxide

You'll find the relevant section at the end of the final paragraph. 'Oil' is mentioned twice in the final paragraph, and the second time, there is a clear agreement between the statement and passage: 'For years, oil companies have taken carbon dioxide from underground deposits... to aid in flushing oil from dwindling reservoirs.'

Set 7

1. Psychology was first studied in Ancient Greece.

Question: Which of the following statements is least likely to be true? (i.e. most likely to be false or can't tell).

Note that 'least likely to be true' means you're not just looking for a false statement - a correct statement could also be 'Can't tell' if it's the least likely to be true out of all the options.

A: Hippocrates proposed that disorders of the mind had a physical origin.

Keywords: Hippocrates, physical, disorders

It is best to scan for a name, in this case 'Hippocrates', which leads us to the end of the first paragraph. The passage directly echoes the question statement: 'mental disorders were of a physical... nature'. Thus, this statement is true. Discard.

B: Psychoanalysis is a dated form of psychotherapy.

Keywords: Psychoanalysis, psychotherapy, dated

'Psychoanalysis' and its role in 'psychotherapy' clearly play important parts in this statement: we can find both these keywords in the third paragraph. The passage reveals 'psychoanalysis 'to be contrasted with 'newer, more widely used psychotherapies' - thus, this is consistent with the question statement and so discard.

C: Watson is credited with the establishment of behaviourism.

Keywords: Watson, behaviourism

Again, names are great to skim for: we find 'Watson' in the last paragraph, and the sentence containing this keyword states that 'behaviourism' was a discipline that was 'established... by John Watson', therefore agreeing with the statement. Discard, and move on to the next question: it is important not to waste time checking remaining answer options even if you're only semi-confident in your answer; you have less time to tackle these questions in comparison to true/false/can't tell questions, so it is vital to learn to be ruthless when discarding and move quickly.

D: Psychology was first studied in Ancient Greece.

Keywords: Greece, Psychology

The keyword 'Greece', alongside the more common keyword 'Psychology', brings us to the very first sentence, which does not indicate psychology to have been studied in full sense of the discipline in Ancient times, but only in a 'philosophical context'. Although the text states that 'the study of psychology dates back to the ancient civilizations of Egypt, Greece…' we can' tell from this if it was first studied in Ancient Greece. Importantly, there is no mention of Ancient Greece being the 'first' civilization to be involved in the study of Psychology. Thus, this is the answer.

2. Scientific progress in the 19th century played a role in inspiring Wundt to bring the study of Psychology into the experimental realm.

Question: Which of the following statements is true?

> **A: Behavioural tendencies depend upon the generation of pleasant or painful emotions in response to internal stimuli.**

Keywords: Behaviour, pleasant/painful, internal stimuli

Skimming for 'behaviour', as well as 'pleasant/painful' brings us to the last paragraph. The passage makes clear that behavioural tendencies were a result of associations with 'environmental stimuli' opposed to 'internal stimuli'. Thus, this statement is false. Discard.

> **B: Scientific progress in the 19th century played a role in inspiring Wundt to bring the study of Psychology into the experimental realm.**

Keywords: Wundt, 19th century, Scientific progress, Psychology, Experimental

There are quite a few keywords you could use to skim for the relevant part of the passage, but names are always good because the passage won't have synonyms for names: skimming for 'Wundt' takes us to the second paragraph. Reading the corresponding sentence tells us that 'Wundt... was motivated in part by... recent advances in chemistry'; as a result, this may have played a role in the introduction of psychological discovery into an 'experimental setting'. Thus, this statement is true - discard the remaining answer options and move on.

> **C: Behaviourism was established towards the end of the 20th century.**

Keywords: Behaviourism, 20th century, establish

Skimming leads us to the last paragraph, which directly states behaviourism was established in the 'early' 20th century, not towards the end - thus, this statement is false.

> **D: Aristotle played a major role in the foundations underlying psychology today.**

Keywords: Aristotle, foundations, psychology

The only place 'Aristotle' is mentioned is in the first paragraph: there is no mention of him playing any role in the foundations underlying psychology: we need more information, and thus this statement would be classified as 'can't tell'.

3. A behaviourist would argue that our behavioural patterns are guided by rewarding and aversive stimuli.

Question: Which of the following statements can be inferred from the passage?

A: Behaviourist theories still play a prominent role in psychology today.

Keywords: Behaviourist, theory, psychology

By now, you should be much more familiar with the passage: the thing with SBA sets is that although it will be extremely slow to begin with, by the 3rd question you should have a fuller picture of what the passage is talking about, as well as knowing where things are. Although it was 'dominant in the 1950s', there is no mention of behaviourist theories playing a prominent role in psychology today,

B: A behaviourist would argue that our behavioural patterns are guided by rewarding and aversive stimuli.

Keywords: Behaviourist, patterns, stimuli

This statement also takes us to the final paragraph. We know that 'behavioural tendencies' are determined by associations between 'stimuli' and the degree of 'pleasure or pain' that follows. In other words, rewards, which induce pleasure, and aversive stimuli that bring about unpleasant sensations, would naturally be implicated in the development of behavioural patterns and likely needed for guiding such actions. Discard the remaining answer options and move on.

C: Behaviourist theories were influenced by Freud's experimental work during the early 20th century.

Keywords: Behaviourist, Freud, 20th century

There is no mention of 'Freud' playing any role in the behaviourist theories that arose around the same time. Thus, this statement requires information that is not within the passage.

D: A conditioned response to external stimuli is sufficient to produce behavioural patterns.

Keywords: Conditioned, external stimuli, behavioural patterns

Although 'behavioural patterns' involved organisms' conditioned responses to environmental stimuli, this does not indicate it is 'sufficient' to induce behaviour. Thus, this statement is can't tell.

4. Therapists offering Cognitive Analytical Therapy require subjects to undergo therapy at least once a month.

Question: Which of the following statements is false?

A: Psychoanalysis has been proposed to be able to resolve unconscious conflict.

Keywords: Psychoanalysis, unconscious conflict

This is in direct agreement with the passage, near the middle of the second paragraph, with psychoanalysis being thought to 'treat psychological or emotional distress, especially unconscious conflict'.

B: Therapists offering Cognitive Analytical Therapy require subjects to undergo therapy once a month.

Keywords: Cognitive Analytical Therapy, Laboratory

Skimming for 'Cognitive Analytical Therapy' brings us to the end of the third paragraph, which clearly states that such psychotherapies require the 'subject to see their therapist once a week'. This is in direct disagreement with the question statement: thus, this statement is false - discard the remaining options.

C: Wundt established the first psychological laboratory.

Keywords: Wundt, Psychological laboratory

This is in direct agreement with the second paragraph: 'Wundt... founded the first psychological laboratory'.

D: Sigmund Freud died in 1939.

Keywords: 1939, Freud

The best keyword to skim for is '1939', leading us to the beginning of the first sentence of the third paragraph, which clearly states that Freud died during this year. Thus, this statement is true.

Set 8

1. Genetic maturation and environmental factors both have an influence on the psychological development of children.

Question: According to the passage, which of the following statements best apply to a child's development?

Keyword: Psychological development (1st paragraph)

A: From birth, there are intervals, or pauses, in a child's psychological development.

Keywords: Intervals/Pauses

The first paragraph tells us a child's psychological development is a 'continuous process'. Therefore, the statement contradicts the passage.

B: Psychological development is not dependent on the mother.

Keywords: Mother

There is no mention of the keyword 'mother'. Immediately discard - the statement is most likely 'Can't tell'.

C: Genetic maturation and environmental factors both have an influence on the psychological development of children.

Keywords: Genetic, Maturation, Environmental

The first paragraph tells us a child develops 'under the influence of genetic and environmental factors. As a result, this statement agrees with the passage.

D: Psychological development is linked inherently with emotional changes.

Keywords: Emotional

Although both the keywords 'Emotional' and 'Psychological' appear in the first paragraph, there isn't enough information in the passage to draw a link between the two. Discard.

2. Hearing impairment

Question: Which of the following is a common cause of language delay, according to the passage?

Keywords: Language delay (last paragraph). Scan for language delay in the paragraph.

A: Cerebral Infarction

Keywords: Cerebral Infarction

This keyword doesn't appear anywhere in the passage - therefore discard and move on.

B: Autism

Keywords: Autism

Autism causes delays 'occasionally' - this suggests it's not a common cause - discard. Do not overthink.

C: Auditory processing disorders

Keywords: Auditory processing disorders

Again, auditory processing disorders causes delays only occasionally, so discard.

D: Hearing impairment

Keywords: Hearing impairment

The passage states hearing impairment is 'one of the most common causes of language delay'. Therefore, this is the correct answer.

3. No children under the age of 12 months have the ability to use expressive language.

Question: According to the passage, which of the following is least likely to be true?

A: During development, a child's maturation is due to genetically controlled processes.

Keywords: Maturation, Genetically controlled

The passage directly agrees with this statement near the end of the first paragraph.

B: Newborns do not appear to have a fear response.

Keywords: Fear, Newborns

The passage agrees with this statement (in the second paragraph).

C: No children under the age of 12 months have the ability to use expressive language.

Keywords: 12 months, Expressive language

The passage explicitly states expressive language 'begins around 12 months'. The use of the word 'around' suggests some children under the age of 12 months can use expressive language. The use of an absolute word ('no') in the statement makes it even more unlikely. This is therefore the correct answer.

D: Newborns are not able to smile in a social context until around 6 weeks of age.

Keywords: 6 weeks, smile

At the beginning of the first paragraph, the passage states the first learnt social interaction is the 'smile', which starts at about 6 weeks of age'. This is a direct agreement, so can't be untrue.

4. A child is able to produce longer sentences around 3 years of age.

Question: Which of the following, regarding the understanding of speech, is most likely correct, according to the passage?

Keywords: Speech, Understanding

A: The use of expressive language begins to increase quickly around 15 month's age.

Keywords: 15 months, Expressive language

There is no use of the keyword '15 months', so we can immediately assume the statement is False or Can't Tell. On further skimming, the passage states expressive language 'accelerates rapidly' at 18 months. This contradicts the statement.

B: A child can produce longer sentences around 3 years of age.

Keywords: 3 years of age, longer sentences

The keyword '3 years' appears in the third paragraph - the passage tells us that by this time, a child can 'produce complex sentences. This agrees with the statement.

C: A child is unable to produce three worded sentences at 2 years of age.

Keywords: 2 years, three worded sentences

The passage clearly states, in the third paragraph, a child is able to produce 'three or four worded sentences... by 2 years of age.'. This contradicts the statement.

D: It would take at least 6 years for most children to be able to produce any language similar to that of an adult.

Keywords: 6 years, Adult

In the third paragraph, we can see that that it takes '5 years' for a child to be able to use language in similar ways to an adult. This statement is 'false'.

Set 9

1. Blue whales sometimes feed on other things aside from Zooplankton.

Question: The passage supports which of the following conclusions?

A: Krill descend during the day and come to the surface at night.

Keywords: Krill, Surface

You'll find the relevant passage halfway through the second passage by skimming for 'Krill'. Although blue whales hunt krill in this pattern (descending during the day and surfacing at night), there could be other explanations for this movement. Don't make assumptions without sufficient evidence.

B: The blue whale is the largest animal that has ever existed.

Keywords: Blue whale

The keyword 'Blue Whale' can be found at the beginning of the first paragraph. The largest animal that has ever existed' is a bold statement. Although the passage does claim the blue whale is the largest known animal that has existed, this does not rule out animals that have not yet been discovered. The statement is beyond the passage.

> C: Bowhead whale population drastically decreased due to commercial whaling in the 19th century.

Keywords: 19th Century, Bowhead whale, Commercial whaling

The passage mentions a decrease in the blue world population due to commercial whaling, but Bowhead whales are not included in this section of the passage. This statement is beyond the passage.

> D: Blue whales sometimes feed on other things aside from Zooplankton.

Keywords: Zooplankton, Blue Whales

In the second paragraph, the passage states 'the blue whale… almost exclusively feeds on zooplankton'. The qualifier 'almost' means we can infer Blue whales feed on other things.

2. Krill are a type of Zooplankton.

Question: Using information from the passage, we can infer that:

> A: The whaling ban has had little effect on the blue whale population.

Keywords: Whaling ban, Blue Whale, Population

The keyword 'whaling ban' appears in the last sentence of the last paragraph. There is an estimated increase of 7.3% of the blue whale population every year, therefore, the whaling ban has had an effect on the population of Blue whales. This statement contradicts the passage, so discard.

> B: Krill are a type of Zooplankton.

Keywords: Krill, Zooplankton

'Krill' appears again in the second paragraph. The article states blue whales feed 'almost exclusively' on Zooplankton, and 'eat up to 3600 kg of Krill in a day'. 3600 kg is a significant amount, and so we can infer Krill are a type of Zooplankton.

> C: Female blue whales give birth at least once a month.

Keywords: Birth, Female, Blue Whales, Month

The keyword 'birth' appears in the third paragraph. The passage directly contradicts the statement - female whales give birth every 2-3 months.

> D: Some blue whales are killed by sharks every year.

Keywords: Sharks, Blue Whales

There is no reference of 'sharks' in the passage, therefore the answer will be beyond the passage.

3. Some types of mammal do not produce milk for their young.

Question: Which of the following statements about mammals are false?

Keyword: Mammal

> A: Minke whales are a type of mammal.

Keyword: Minke Whales

The keyword from the question ('mammals') appears at the end of the first paragraph. The extract, 'Like all mammals, whales...', clearly suggests whales are mammals, and therefore, we have a direct agreement. Discard.

B: All whales are warm blooded.

Keywords: Warm blooded

At the end of the first paragraph, the passage directly agrees with this statement.

C: Like monkeys, whales have body hair.

Keywords: Body hair

The passage explicitly states, 'all' mammals have 'body hair'- therefore discard.

D: Some types of mammal do not produce milk for their young.

Keywords: milk, (mammal)

By eliminating all the other options (and from the passage), this must be the correct answer.

4. The population of all types of whale in the suborder Mysticeti was reduced by whaling.

Question: Referring to the passage, all of these statements are likely to be true, except...

A: Due to their size, blue whales have few natural predators.

Keywords: Natural predators, Blue whales

The keyword 'natural predator' appears at the end of the second paragraph. There are 'virtually' no natural predators' because 'blue whales themselves are so large', therefore the passage contradicts the statement. Discard.

B: Whales can reproduce 9 years from birth after having reached sexual maturity.

Keywords: 9 years, Sexual maturity

'Sexual maturity' (third paragraph) is reached in about '7 years'. We can therefore infer whales can reproduce 9 years from birth. Discard.

C: The population of all the different types of whales in the suborder Mysticeti was reduced by whaling.

Keywords: Mysticeti, Whaling

Once again, the keyword 'whaling' is found in the last paragraph, and only 'blue whales' are specifically mentioned. There is no information on other types of whale and if they were affected by hunting. The statement is therefore beyond the passage and least likely to be true.

D: Bowhead whales could potentially live more than 100 years.

Keywords: 100 years, Bowhead whales

'100 years' appears at the end of the third paragraph. The passage tells us total lifespan could be 'over 100 years'. Although not proven, there is certainly a potential for this to be the case as the passage suggests.

1. Males accounted for roughly 5,600 alcohol-related deaths in the UK in 2012.

Question: Using information in the passage, the writer would probably most agree with which one of the following?

A: Alcohol accounts for approximately 400,000 hospital admissions in the UK.

Keywords: 400,000, hospital admissions, UK

Numbers and abbreviations are great keywords to skim for - and although there is no direct reference to '400,000', our eyes are immediately drawn to the last paragraph. Do expect basic maths during VR, although this represents a very small proportion of questions. We know that alcohol accounts for 6% of all hospital admissions, but we don't know the total number of admissions - thus, we don't have enough information in the passage to support this statement.

B: Both male and female prisoners on average report drinking 200 units a month.

Keywords: 200 units, prisoners

The relevant part of the passage is found in the last paragraph: we know that prisoners drink an average of '20 units a day', but this does not translate to 200 units a month; it gives instead a monthly average of roughly 600 units. Thus, this statement is false.

C: Males accounted for roughly 5,600 alcohol-related deaths in the UK in 2012.

Keywords: 5,600, alcohol-related deaths, UK, 2012, Males

By now, it should be clear that all statistical information within the passage is in the last paragraph. '70%' of all alcohol-related deaths in 2012 were male, and there were '8,000' alcohol-related deaths in total. An easy way of finding this percentage of the total is by first taking 10% of 8,000, which is 800, and then multiplying it by 7: 800 x 7 = 5,600. This is in agreement with the statement and therefore true. Select and discard remaining options.

D: There are around 1.5 million violent incidents a year.

Keywords: 1.5 million, violent incidents

The last paragraph states that 'roughly half of all reported violent incidents in a year 'were by offenders under the influence of alcohol, which represented 900,000 cases. The total number of violent incidents should therefore be double this number: 1.8 million violent offenses. This is inconsistent with the statement and therefore false.

2. The alleviation of withdrawal symptoms is not common reason for continuing drinking habits amongst alcoholics.

Question: Which of the following statements is FALSE?

A: Limiting access to alcohol can play a part in reducing alcoholism.

Keywords: Access to alcohol, alcoholism

We find that 'inexpensive easily accessible alcohol' increases risk - and also that prevention of alcoholism is possible by limiting the sale of alcohol. Therefore, this statement agrees with the passage.

B: The alleviation of withdrawal symptoms is not common reason for continuing drinking habits amongst alcoholics.

Keywords: Withdrawal, Drinking/Alcoholics

The keyword 'withdrawal' is used first at the end of the first paragraph, but does not make a reference to continuing drinking habits; the end of the second paragraph, however, directly disagrees with this statement, where alcoholics 'typically continue to drink' partly to prevent or improve symptoms of withdrawal. Hence, this statement is false and the correct answer for this question.

C: The increasing numbers of young offenders may be a result of corresponding increases in alcohol consumption amongst young people.

Keywords: young offenders, alcohol consumption, young people

Although crime is mentioned in the last paragraph, the concept of 'young offenders' and 'young people' do not appear anywhere in the passage. Thus, we cannot tell if this statement is true or not based on the information in the passage.

D: Treatment for alcoholics is not always a simple, single-step process.

Keywords: Treatment, simple/single-step process

Skimming for 'treatment' brings us to the beginning of the third paragraph, which states that treatment may take 'several steps'. This agrees with the statement, and hence it is true.

3. Group or self-help therapy is necessary for preventing a return to alcohol dependency.

Question: According to the passage, the author would LEAST likely agree with which one of the following?

A: A person with trouble reducing alcohol consumption and who cannot fulfil day-to-day responsibilities due to such usage can be termed alcoholic.

Keywords: reduction alcohol, responsibilities, alcoholic

The relevant part of the passage can be found in the first paragraph, where alcoholism is said to exist when two of several criteria are met, including 'usage resulting in failure to fulfil responsibilities' and 'difficulty cutting down'. Thus, this is in agreement with the statement.

B: Many of the factors leading to and causing alcoholism are out of a person's control.

Keywords: alcoholism, control

This question is more difficult because there are few keywords to latch onto. However, the second paragraph makes it clear that several factors contribute to alcoholism, half of which are genetic, which confirms that many factors are not in a subject's control. Moreover, environmental factors, such as social or cultural issues, are not always easily controllable.

C: Rapid, uncontrolled detoxification in alcoholics can lead to serious health complications.

Keywords: detoxification, health complications, alcoholics

Skimming for 'detoxification', we find it in the third paragraph, which makes it clear that 'detoxification should be carefully controlled' and in order to prevent the 'severe' medical problems that can occur during withdrawal. The passage thus agrees with the statement.

> **D: Group or self-help therapy is necessary for preventing a return to alcohol dependency.**

Keywords: Group/Self-help therapy, alcoholism/dependency

'Group' or 'self-help therapy' is mentioned at the end of the third paragraph, where the passage tells us that these are used to 'help keep a person from returning to drinking'. It does not, however, indicate that it is 'necessary' for the prevention of alcohol dependency, and so goes beyond what can be inferred or gained from the passage. Thus, this is the correct answer.

4. The risk of alcoholism can be 400% higher for a person with an alcoholic sibling.

Question: Which of the following is true?

> **A: Increased pricing of alcohol will not act as a deterrent for alcoholics.**

Keywords: pricing, deterrent, alcoholics

The third paragraph states that 'taxing alcohol to increase its cost' may help in preventing alcoholism. Thus, this statement does not agree with the passage: moreover, it uses bold language - 'will not' - and so should give an immediate clue of its questionable validity.

> **B: The risk of alcoholism can be 400% higher for a person with an alcoholic sibling.**

Keywords: 400%, sibling

'400%' is not present in the passage, but may require some kind of derivation; indeed, skimming for 'sibling' brings us to the beginning of the second paragraph, where the passage states a person with a sibling who is alcoholic are three to four times as likely to become alcoholic themselves. 'Four times' is equivalent to '400%', and so the statement is true.

> **C: Stress and anxiety play little part as factors leading to alcoholism.**

Keywords: Stress/Anxiety, alcoholism

The second paragraph directly states that 'high stress levels' and 'anxiety' increases risk of alcoholism. Hence, this statement is false.

> **D: There are more young people than adults committing alcohol-related crimes.**

Keywords: young people/adults, alcohol-related crimes

Again, although crime is discussed in the last paragraph, 'young people' are not mentioned anywhere in the passage and certainly not a comparison between young offenders and adult offenders. Thus, evaluation of this statement required further information not included in the passage.

41. The Cosmic rays recorded near the surface of the earth tend to be high energy particles.

Question: According to the passage, which of the following is the most likely to be true?

A: All charged particles in interplanetary space originate from the sun.

Keywords: Interplanetary space, Sun

The keyword 'interplanetary space' leads us to the first line. We can see it's a clear contradiction: 'not all the charged particles in interplanetary space come from the sun'. Be wary of the use of absolute language (such as 'all', 'always', etc.) in statements.

B: Cosmic rays are slow moving particles that enter the atmosphere.

Keywords: Cosmic rays, Slow moving particles, Atmosphere

The keyword 'Cosmic rays' appears in the first paragraph, and after examining the context, the passage tells us 'high-speed intruders... as they bombard the atmosphere' were named cosmic rays. This contradicts the statement, so discard.

C: Removing electrons from an atom can be achieved by accelerating it to near the speed of light.

Keywords: Speed of light, Accelerating, Electrons, Atom

'Speed of light' brings us to the second sentence of the first paragraph. We can see the passage doesn't suggest a relationship, and as a result, the statement is beyond the passage.

D: The Cosmic rays recorded near the surface of the earth tend to be high energy particles.

Keywords: High energy particles, Cosmic rays, Surface, Earth

The keyword 'energy' leads us to the first paragraph. The passage tells us the 'more energetic fraction of these particles bombard the atmosphere' - this suggests the rays near the surface of the earth have higher energy. To further confirm this, near the end of the first paragraph, the statement 'rays with lower energies than those recorded near the surface of Earth...' also suggests rays near the surface of the earth tend to be at a higher energy level.

2. A magnetic field carried by solar wind outflow which distorts the path of incoming rays.

Question: Which of the following is the best reason cosmic rays are prevented from fully penetrating the sun, according to the passage?

Keywords: Cosmic rays, Penetration, Sun

A: There is a strong 'surf' of UV rays, from the solar wind, that diverts incoming rays.

Keywords: UV Rays, Solar Wind

Skimming the passage, we can't find any mention of the keyword 'UV Rays'. Instead, magnetic waves are the only type of wave that's stated in the passage. Discard this statement.

B: Solar wind outflow directly acts as an obstacle to cosmic rays.

Keywords: Solar wind outflow, Obstacle

The 'lack of collision' between cosmic rays and solar-wind particles (found around the middle of the second paragraph) is due to the 'low densities of material'. We can infer the particles are probably quite small and does not play much of a role in preventing cosmic rays penetrating the sun. Therefore, this statement makes a contradictory inference.

C: A magnetic field carried by solar wind outflow which distorts the path of incoming rays.

Keywords: Magnetic field, Solar wind outflow

The passage states, in the second paragraph, 'after the solar wind leaves the vicinity of the sun... it carries part of the solar magnetic field along with it...'. As a result, 'incoming rays are subject to the forces that magnetic fields exert...' The passage also tells us this is a 'barrier', and, therefore, this statement is true.

D: An abundance of low density material in 'empty space'

Keywords: Low density material, Empty space. Low density material results in a 'lack of collision' - this statement is false.

3. Coronal holes can be found over the poles of the sun.

Question: Which of the following would the author most agree with?

A: It is equally difficult for cosmic rays to penetrate the heliosphere.

Keywords: Heliosphere

The relevant section can be found near the beginning of the final paragraph. The passage tells us 'cosmic rays traveling inward over the poles of the sun might penetrate the heliosphere more easily'. This directly contradicts the statement.

B: Coronal holes can be found over the poles of the sun.

Keywords: Coronal holes, Poles, Sun

The final paragraph states cosmic rays may penetrate the heliosphere easier if they travel inward over the 'poles of the sun'. A reason for this occurrence was the comparatively smoother flow of solar wind from 'coronal holes'. We can reasonably infer from this information coronal holes can be found over the poles of the sun

C: Charged particles don't follow a distinct path along magnetic field lines.

Keywords: Charged, Magnetic field lines

The final paragraph tells us 'charged particles' follow a helical path along magnetic field lines – this contradicts the statement.

D: The lines of force connecting with the poles of the sun are weak channels for cosmic rays to penetrate the sun.

Keywords: Poles of the sun, Channel

The passage clearly states the lines of force connecting with the poles are excellent conduits into the inner heliosphere, and so the passage contradicts the statement.

4. The heliosphere surrounds the sun.

Question: According to the passage, which of the following is most likely to be true?

A: The heliosphere surrounds the sun.

Keywords: Heliosphere

From the context of the final paragraph, it strongly suggests the heliosphere surrounds the sun: 'cosmic rays... traveling over the poles of the sun might penetrate the heliosphere'. This statement is likely to be true.

B: Cosmic rays can only be measured by people in spacecraft.

Keywords: Spacecraft

The relevant section can be found in the first paragraph. Although the earliest spacecraft measurements of cosmic rays were obtained four decades ago, the same paragraph also tells us 'Earthbound researchers' have been able to measure particles. The passage contradicts the statement.

C: Solar wind is caused by a similar mechanism controlling wind on Earth.

Keywords: Solar wind

There is no mention of wind on Earth, nor its mechanism - this statement is beyond the passage.

D: Most cosmic rays penetrate the inner heliosphere.

Keywords: Heliosphere

The relevant section is near the beginning of the second paragraph. The passage clearly states 'only a portion' of cosmic rays penetrate the inner heliosphere, and so it directly contradicts the statement.

Decision Making

What is 'Decision Making'?

The Decision Making section was introduced in 2017 to replace the old Decision Analysis section. The old version was thought to be too easy and artificially inflated scores. The new section revolves around testing three main aspects: evaluating arguments, using deductive reasoning, and interpreting statistics & figures.

Lots of the questions ask you to decide which conclusions do and do not follow logically from a passage. Others give you a statement and ask you to select the strongest argument in its favour. It is important for a clinician to be able to quickly draw conclusions from information they have been given and evaluate the strength of arguments, ensuring that they are not misled by their own beliefs. The statistical and figurative reasoning questions assess a candidate's ability to interpret Set Theory, whether it is in the form of text or Venn diagrams, and their ability to evaluate probability.

Why do you have to do DM?

Doctors and dentists frequently encounter complex situations which require quick and accurate problem solving. This section is designed to assess how logical a candidate is in their thought process, especially under pressure.

Although this section is designed to be more difficult to prepare for and to test more of the candidate's natural decision making abilities than the old Decision Analysis section, there remain a number of ways to boost your performance.

Numbers for this section

- **Time**

  32 minutes total = 1 minute for instructions + 31 minutes to complete

- **Questions**

  29 questions total

  Some items may include multiple parts

  6 questions types

  - Syllogisms
  - Logic Puzzles
  - Interpreting Information
  - Recognising Assumptions
  - Probability
  - Venn Diagrams

Timing for this section will be varied with some questions taking a lot of time and others taking much less and so as with other sections you will have to make up time in the easier questions to be able to use more time in the harder questions. There is no relationship between the questions, so each question will take time to read and understand.

Question Types

As mentioned before there are 3 main aspects being tested each with their question types. Each question type covers a different skill and has a very different approach. Below are some examples of each question type.

Deductive Reasoning	Evaluating Arguments	Figure Analysis
- Syllogisms	- Interpreting Information	- Probability
- Logical Puzzles	- Recognising Assumptions	- Venn Diagrams

There is a fairly even emphasis placed on the 3 domains of questions, with approximately 10 or 11 questions each for the deductive reasoning and evaluating arguments domains and approximately 9 questions for the figure analysis domain. However, this may vary between each examination.

There are 2 main formats of questions in this section; the first where you have to choose the single best answer from 4 options, and the second where you have to evaluate 5 statements and mark them yes or no. Unlike previous section, each question is standalone and questions are not arranged in 'sets' on similar themes. The marking for this second type of question reflects the extra work required, by giving full credit to a candidate that evaluates all 5 statements correctly, but importantly also awards partial credit if a candidate assesses some but not all the statements correctly.

Preparation Tips

1. Practice as you mean to go on

For most, this section requires significant use of the whiteboard and pen, so make sure you practise with a similar set-up. It's important, when using the whiteboard so much, to keep your work organised so you don't waste time looking for an answer you already have. While it's important to write down important information, practice only writing down the information that is necessary in order to maximise your efficiency.

2. Focus on keeping it simple

It's important to keep it simple in this section - answer the questions using only the information you have in front of you. It's easy to bring in outside knowledge without realising, but a good clinician avoids making assumptions based on information they don't have. Focus on what the question is asking you, some of the information may just be there to waste your time.

3. Guess, Flag, Skip

This is another section where you will need to triage and work out which questions will take up more time than is appropriate, and employ the guess, flag, skip method. The most difficult questions are those involving multiple statements or complicated Venn diagrams, but as you practice you may find that other question types are more time-consuming for you, and choose to guess, flag and skip those instead.

Syllogisms

Approach

In a syllogism question, you will be given a series of premises. You will then need to use deductive reasoning to determine whether a conclusion does or does not follow.

For example:

Premise 1: All windows are made from glass

Premise 2: All glass is made from sand

Inferred Conclusion: All windows are made from sand

You will notice that syllogisms follow a simple form of:

Premise 1: A → B

Premise 2: B → C

Inferred Conclusion: A → C

Using this form, it is possible to break down the premises to their most basic parts and more easily see a link, if any, between the 2 premises.

N.B. It's important to realise that the premises work in one direction only. For example, a statement that says 'All the shoppers were male' can be written as All Shoppers → Male, but not as All Males → Shoppers.

Here's the **three-step approach** you should take for syllogism questions:

1. Evaluate the premises
2. Link the premises
3. Answer the question

And, as always, here's the approach in more detail:

Step 1: Evaluate the premises

Begin by making yourself familiar with the premises in the question and break it down into its constituent parts if necessary. This is done by identifying the key words in the statement and replacing the rest with arrows to demonstrate the relationships between these ideas. For example, a statement that reads:

'All taxi drivers drive black cabs; some black cabs have 6 seats' can be broken down to:

All Taxi Drivers → Drive Black Cabs

Some Black Cabs → 6 seats

Step 2: Link the premises

This requires you to draw a conclusion from the separate premises to produce a single simplified statement, remembering to consider the qualifiers and absolutes in the text. For example, if a statement uses the word all you must include this in the premise and conclusions. For example, from the premises we looked at above, we can thus conclude that:

Some Taxi Drivers → 6 seats

Step 3: Answer the question

Now you should go through each of the questions in turn and work out whether you can draw the conclusion given with only the information above. Remember to avoid bringing in your own knowledge as this may result in you incorrectly marking answers. For example, can you draw the conclusion: Some black cabs have fewer than 6 seats?

Answer: No, while we know that some cabs have a different number of seats there is no information provided on whether the other cabs have fewer or a greater number of seats.

Walkthrough

We're going to take you through the 3-step method by applying it to the following question:

"All fish that have scales can swim. Kurilian Bobtails are unable to swim."

Circle 'Yes' if the conclusion does follow. Circle 'No' if the conclusion does not follow.

Kurilian Bobtails are a type of fish.	Yes/No
Kurilian Bobtails are not a type of fish.	Yes/No
Kurilian Bobtails have scales.	Yes/No
Given that a Kurilian Bobtail is a type of fish, it does not have scales.	Yes/No
Sharks can swim	Yes/No

The first step is to evaluate the premises. We can break down the premises into their basic parts:

All fish that have scales can swim

All fish with scales ⇒ Swim

Kurilian Bobtails are unable to swim

Kurilian Bobtails ⇏ Swim

Having broken down the premises, the next step is to link the premises. In this case, it can seen that there is no easy direct link, but we can be sure that because the Kurilian Bobtail is unable to swim that it is not a fish with scales, and thus rewrite the 2 premises into this single conclusion:

It's now time to answer the questions.

Kurilian Bobtail's are a type of fish. Yes/**No**

From the original premises and conclusion we have drawn, we only know that Kurilian Bobtails are definitely not fish with scales. They could be a non-swimming fish without scales or not a fish at all.

Kurilian Bobtail's are not a type of fish. Yes/**No**

Similar to the previous question, all we know is that Kurilian Bobtails are definitely not fish with scales. They could be a non-swimming fish without scales or not a fish at all. We cannot say that this conclusion follows.

Kurilian Bobtail's have scales. Yes/**No**

While we cannot rule out the possibility that Kurilian Bobtails are a non-fish with scales, we do not have enough information to conclude this.

Given that a Kurilian Bobtail is a type of fish, it does not have scales. **Yes**/No

This conclusion gives us more information, which we should evaluate. Seeing as we know that all fish with scales can swim, we are certain the Kurilian Bobtail is not a fish with scales. Therefore, given that it is a fish, it would have to be a fish without scales.

Sharks can swim Yes/**No**

This conclusion is trying to make us use outside information. Nothing in the question supports this conclusion, so we must answer no.

Qualifiers and Absolutes

Similar to the Verbal Reasoning section, you need to consider the qualifiers and absolutes in the premises to be able to decide whether a conclusion can be drawn or not. An absolute in one premise must be matched in another premise for a valid conclusion to be drawn. Below are a few of the most common examples of qualifiers and absolutes you will come across, but note that all of these have some exceptions.

All + All = All

All tigers are felines, all felines have claws

Therefore, we can conclude that all tigers have claws

All + Some = Insufficient

All tigers are felines, some felines have claws

We cannot conclude that all tigers have claws, that no tigers have claws, or some tigers have claws.

All + No = No

All tigers are felines, no felines have claws

Therefore, we can conclude that all tigers do not have claws

Some + All = Some

Some boats are tankers, all tankers carry oil

Therefore, we can conclude that some boats carry oil

Some + Some = Insufficient

Some boats are tankers, some tankers carry oil

We cannot conclude that some boats carry oil. For example, the tankers that carry oil might be on-land tankers and therefore not be boats. Remember, you cannot bring in outside knowledge.

Some + No = Some No

Some boats are tankers, no tankers carry oil

Therefore, some boats do not carry oil.

No + All = Insufficient

No houses have fences, all fences have spikes

Therefore, we cannot conclude that the houses don't have spikes, or that houses do have spikes, as we don't have enough information

No + Some = Insufficient

No houses have fences, some fences have spikes

Therefore, like before, we need more information before we can draw a conclusion.

No + No = Insufficient

No houses have fences, no fences have spikes

Therefore, we need more information before we can draw a link between houses and spikes.

Logic Puzzles

Approach

In this section you will have to use the information given to deduce the correct answer option.

Here's the **three-step approach** you should take for logical puzzle questions:

1. Read the statement and question
2. Create a table
3. Discard and Decide

And here is the method in more detail:

Step 1: Read the statement and question

Identify the main subjects and other variables in the statement to help you with the next step. Similar to the other question types, reading the question and answer options is important to avoid wasting time working out more information than is necessary. Some questions will be more straightforward and will not require a table.

Step 2: Create a table

Tables are quick to create and allow us to visualise the information from the statement. Write down the main subjects in the first column and refer back to the statements to complete the other columns. There may be multiple spaces you can't fill, but this may not be necessary to complete the question, so don't waste time.

Step 3: Discard and Decide

Using the table, you have created, go through each of the answer options one by one and decide whether it follows from the information given in the statement.

Walkthrough

We're going to take you through the 3-step method by applying it to the following question:

In a Formula 1 race there are 6 people competing. Ross finishes last after starting the race one position higher. Rachel finishes in the position Monica started the race on. Joey finishes one place behind Chandler, who started in second place. Monica started the race ahead of Chandler but ended up one place ahead of Ross. Phoebe started fourth but finished ahead of Chandler.

Who ended the race in fourth place?

A. Rachel   B. Chandler   C. Joey   D. Phoebe

The first step is to read the statement and question briefly to get a good idea of what we need to work out. From the statement, we can identify that the main characters are Ross, Rachel, Monica, Joey, Chandler and Phoebe. We can also tell that the two pieces of information that might be important are the starting position and the finishing position.

From the question, we can see that the most important piece of information is the fourth place finishing position, so once we've worked out this information, we know we can answer the question.

It's now time to create a table. From the information we are given, the table should have a column for the racing drivers, a column for the starting position and a column for the finishing position - but the simpler the better! So something like this is great:

	Starting	Finishing
Ross		
Rachel		
Monica		
Joey		
Chandler		
Phoebe		

We now need to use the information given to fill in the spaces as quickly as possible. We know that Ross finishes in 6th position and started one position higher, 5th position, so we can note this down. We cannot do anything with the information about Rachel yet, so we simply move on and come back to her later if necessary.

The next sentence provides two pieces of good information, as we can record that Chandler started the race in 2nd place, as well as the fact that Joey and Chandler finish in consecutive positions. As Monica started ahead of Chandler, she must have started on 1st position. As she finished ahead of Ross, she must have finished in 5th place. Now we can go back to Rachel, and as she finished the same position Monica started in, she must have finished 1st.

Having done all this, we still don't have enough information to answer the question so we must continue, with the sentence about Phoebe which tells us she came ahead of Chandler. This tells us that Phoebe, Chandler and Joey finish in this order and therefore, Joey is the one that finishes 4th. We can therefore select 'C - Joey' as the correct answer.

	Starting	Finishing
Ross	5	6
Rachel		1
Monica	1	5
Joey		4
Chandler	2	3
Phoebe	4	2

Interpreting Information

Approach

With this type of question, you will have to draw a conclusion from the data given in the form of passages, graphs, tables or charts. Some questions may bear similarity to the Quantitative Reasoning section, but questions in this section require fewer calculations. Instead, most of the conclusions you will need to make will come from either eyeballing the data or a very basic calculation (it is unlikely you will need to use the calculator).

Here's the **two-step approach** you should take for interpreting information questions:

Step 1: Look at the data

Don't be afraid if the data looks a little daunting. Take the first few moments to read any titles, axes or keys that may be present and get an idea of what the data is trying to tell you. This is important as it will not only let you know where to find the information you might need, but possibly save you time by stopping you from spending time on working out information you already have. The conclusions below may help you understand the information better as well. If you are still struggling to understand the data, guess, flag and skip!

Step 2: Evaluate conclusions

In this step, you go through each of the conclusions and decide whether they can be drawn from the information above. You don't have to go in order, so you can start on whichever conclusion looks easiest to assess. Remember, this section isn't here to test your maths so you can round most of the figures if needs be. Again, it's important to not judge the conclusions based on how plausible they sound, but instead on how well they are supported from the data.

Walkthrough

We're going to take you through the 2-step method by applying it to the following question:

The profits of 4 companies, Stark Industries, iRobot Inc, Khal Air and Macrosoft are being compared.

Decide whether the following conclusions follow from the graph:

- A. Macrosoft's profits have always increased year-on-year
- B. iRobot has been consistent in its profits
- C. Khal Air is a better company today than in 2012
- D. Stark's profits are always better than most of the other companies.

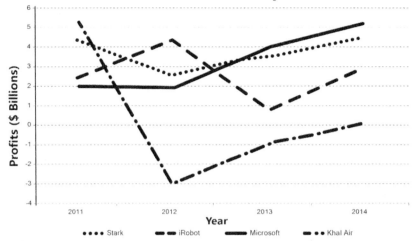

Market Share Companies

The first step is to look at the data. In this case, we are looking at a 4 year period 2011 - 2014, and the profits in billions of dollars. It is important to note that some companies had negative profits (i.e. made a loss) in this time period.

Having familiarised ourselves with the data, we can move onto evaluating the conclusions.

A. Macrosoft's profits have always increased year-on-year

Looking at the graph, we can see that Macrosoft has never decreased its profits year on year, however this is different than the claim that it has increased year on year. In 2012, the profit was the same as in 2011 and thus we cannot say the conclusion is valid.

B. iRobot has been consistent in its profits

iRobot's profits have always changed considerably from the previous year and thus we must disagree with the conclusion.

C. Khal Air is a better company today than in 2012

This is a tricky statement. While it is true to say Khal Air has made a small profit in 2014 rather than a loss in 2012, we do not have enough information to decide whether it is a 'better company'. We must therefore say we cannot agree with the conclusion.

D. Stark's profits are always better than most of the other companies.

Stark has consistently had the 2nd highest profits year on year compared to the other 3 companies. As there are 3 other companies, we can deduce that most of the companies is anything over 50%, and therefore, it is correct to say Stark's profits are better than most of the other companies and agree with this conclusion.

Recognising Assumptions

Approach

In this question type, you are provided with a statement then asked to select the strongest argument, which could be for or against. This tests your scientific thinking, because you need to find the argument that makes the fewest assumptions.

Here's the **three-step approach** you should take for recognising assumptions questions:

1. Read the statement

2. Evaluate the arguments

3. Discard and Decide

Let's look at this method in more detail:

Step 1: Read the statement

Take time to identify the key theme behind the statement and what the question is aiming to answer. For example, if the statement asks 'Should diesel cars be banned from the road to decrease pollution?', then the main theme is the link between diesel cars and pollution. The strongest arguments will therefore directly discuss this theme, either arguing that banning diesel cars will result in decreased pollution, or that banning cars will not lead to a decrease in pollution.

Step 2: Evaluate the arguments

Read each argument individually and first decide whether it is relevant to the question, by determining whether it involves the key theme. If it does, it is more relevant and more likely to be your answer. Next, evaluate whether the argument makes any unreasonable assumptions. This would be a reason to discard it.

Step 3: Discard and Decide

Having discarded the arguments that are irrelevant or that make assumptions, you now have to decide which is the strongest argument. The more directly the option can argue its point compared to the key theme, the stronger the argument. For example, if you have an argument that says 'Yes, as diesel cars are the biggest polluters of all transport' and if you have an argument that says 'Yes, as diesel cars make more pollution than petrol cars', the first argument is considered stronger as it links to the key theme more directly than the second argument.

Walkthrough

We're going to take you through the 3-step method by applying it to the following question:

Should we decrease the consumption of sugar that we eat by creating a tax on it?

Select the strongest argument from the statements below:

A. Yes, more sugar is being eaten than ever before

B. Yes, if sugary products are more expensive, people will be discouraged from buying them

C. No, this will merely affect the poorest consumers disproportionately and raise prices for those who cannot afford it the most

D. No, educating people in schools is more important

The first step is to read the statement and try and work out the key theme here. From the statement 'should we decrease the consumption of sugar by creating a tax on it?', we can understand that the theme of the question is the link between taxing sugar and any subsequent decrease in sugar consumption.

Now we have a theme, we can evaluate the arguments given:

A) Yes, more sugar is being eaten than ever before

While this argument talks about sugar consumption, there is no link to taxation and whether this measure will be effective or ineffective, and so we can be confident this is not the strongest argument and discard this option.

B) Yes, if sugary products are more expensive, people will be discouraged from buying them

This argument is successful as it discusses the theme of the question and provides a reasonable explanation of the link between taxing and consumption of sugar. While this is a valid conclusion, we should evaluate the other arguments before we conclude it is the strongest.

C) No, this will merely affect the poorest consumers disproportionately and raise prices for those who cannot afford it the most

While this argument discusses taxation of sugar, it does not make any explanation as to whether the taxation will decrease or increase consumption. It is important to remember that even if you agree with the argument, that doesn't necessarily make it the strongest.

D) No, educating people in schools is more important

This is irrelevant to the theme of the question, and we have no idea about the efficacy of teaching at schools, so we can discard this statement. Overall, as there were no stronger arguments than 'B', we can select this as the strongest argument.

Probability

Approach

Here's the **three-step approach** you should take for probability questions:

1. Read the statement
2. Work out the probability
3. Discard and Decide

Let's looks at this approach in greater detail:

Step 1: Read the statement

This is important to pick out key points, specifically information such as the probability of an event occurring, the number of events that occur, and the people involved. There may be other relevant information that you might want to make a note of to speed up any calculations you might need to make.

Step 2: Work out the probability

Read the question and use the information to work out whether the answer is YES or NO. This may be aided by a table, but this isn't needed for a lot of questions. You may need to use your knowledge of the AND rule and the OR rule, but remember mental maths should be sufficient to get to the answer.

Step 3: Discard and Decide

Having discarded half of the options, you now have to decide between the remaining options for the correct reasoning. This should not require any further calculation, but simply expresses the calculation you have already done in a statement.

Walkthrough

We're going to take you through the 3-step method by applying it to the following question:

A prize draw allows the winners to pick their prize out of a bag. At the beginning, there are 10 whistles and 20 smartphones. Andy wants to win a whistle and so is waiting for the chance of winning a whistle to increase. Throughout the day, 8 smartphones and 5 whistles are taken out of the bag.

Has the chance of picking out a whistle for Andy increased when the next winner picks a prize?

A. Yes, it was 1/3 and is now 5/17

B. Yes, it was 1/3 and is now 12/17

C. No, it was 1/3 and is now 12/17

D. No, it was 1/3 and is now 5/17

The first step is to read the statement and try and work out the key pieces of information. From the statement, we can see that there are 2 options, picking out the whistle at the chance of 1/3 and picking out the smartphone at the chance of 2/3, and that this probability changes throughout the day.

The easiest way to work out this probability is to create a table like so:

Whistle	Smartphone	Total
10	20	30
5	8	13
5	12	17

You don't need to waste time writing labels such as before and after unless you think you'll mix up the rows. In the first row, we have the number of prizes before the day, in the middle row, the number of devices taken during the day, and in the last row, we have the number of prizes left at the end.

With this information, we can work out that the probability of getting a whistle at the end of the day is 5/17. It is now time to discard and decide the answer options. Straight away we can remove options 'B' and 'C'. The only question now is whether 1/3 is bigger than 5/17; as 1/3 is the equivalent of 5/15, we can see that 5/17 is smaller than 1/3. Therefore, we can see that the chance of picking out a whistle has decreased, and 'D' is the correct answer.

Venn Diagrams

Approach

Here's the three-step approach you should take for Venn Diagram questions:

1. Read the question
2. Picture the data
3. Discard and Decide

Let's look at this method in more detail:

Step 1: Read the question

Spend the first few moments reading the question and the options, to allow you to understand what you're looking for in the data. Once you have a better idea of what you're looking for, you can avoid spending time on working out information that is not relevant to the question. Some questions may not require you to draw a Venn Diagram at all, so don't do more than you have to!

Step 2: Picture the data

If the data is given in a Venn Diagram form, spend the next 10 seconds understanding what the diagram shows. If the data is not in a Venn diagram form, you should guess, flag and skip the question as drawing the diagram can take a lot of time, which you can hopefully accumulate and use at the end.

When you come back to this question later, you should first convert the data into a Venn Diagram. Make sure to use clear labels and a good size diagram that is readable. It might help to identify and write down 2 main things before you start:

1. The categories
2. The total sum of items ($\sum$)

Start with the information that doesn't require any extra working to add to your diagram. Bear in mind that you may not be able to fully complete the Venn diagram, so don't waste too much time if you're stuck.

Step 3: Discard and Decide

Once you have the data in a Venn diagram; keep comparing the options to the diagram, eliminate wrong options, and you should be able to get to the correct answer fairly quickly.

Walkthrough

We're going to take you through the 3-step method by applying it to the following question (with some space for you to draw your own Venn diagram before we ruin the surprise for you!):

A local fish and chip shop were doing a survey on what people requested on their chips.

People had the choice of salt, vinegar and ketchup and were able to choose to have none, one, two or three of the options on their chips.

37 people were part of the survey.

3 people did not want anything on their chips.

8 people had all three options

24 people in total had salt on their chips.

24 people in total had ketchup on their chips.

16 people in total had vinegar on their chips.

9 people opted for just salt and ketchup

4 people opted for just ketchup and vinegar

How many people had just salt and vinegar?

A. 1

B. 3

C. 4

D. 6

The first step is to read the question and work out what we're looking for. We're interested in the amount of people who have only salt and vinegar on their chips, so once we get this information, we can stop trying to fill in the gaps and move on.

We now need to picture the data. Seeing as we don't have a Venn diagram in this question, we can see that this question is likely to take more time than we have and we should guess, flag and skip this question. When we come back to this question, we should identify the main categories and the total number of items.

The main categories are salt, vinegar and ketchup and the total number of participants is 37. This gives us a diagram that looks like this:

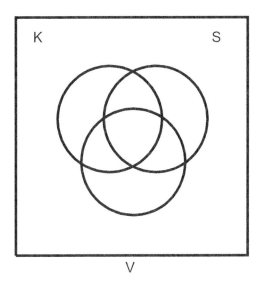

Now we use the information we're given to fill in the gaps, bearing in mind we're mainly interested in the salt category and the vinegar category. 8 people had all 3 toppings, and so we can fill in the middle space. 9 people had just salt and ketchup, and 4 people had just ketchup and vinegar and so we can fill those spaces too. 3 people had nothing on their chips - don't forget to put this number on the outside of your diagram

Seeing as 24 people in total had ketchup on their chips, we can calculate that 3 people had just ketchup. 24 people had salt in total, which means that 7 people had either salt or salt and vinegar; 16 people had vinegar in total, which means that 4 people had either vinegar or salt and vinegar. As the total number of people who we haven't categorised is 10. This means that there must be only 1 person who had both salt and vinegar and the correct answer is 'A'.

Practice Questions

Syllogisms

1. All Europeans of African descent have dark skin, some individuals with dark skin are vitamin D deficient.

Circle 'Yes' if the conclusion does follow. Circle 'No' if the conclusion does not follow.

All Europeans of African descent are vitamin D deficient	Yes/No
Some Europeans of African descent are vitamin D deficient	Yes/No
No vitamin D deficient European has fair skin	Yes/No
Some vitamin D deficient individuals live in Europe	Yes/No
Some Europeans of African descent have fair skin	Yes/No

2. All soft drinks are sweet. Sweet beverages are artificially coloured. Circle 'Yes' if the conclusion does follow. Circle 'No' if the conclusion does not follow.

All soft drinks are artificially coloured	Yes/No
Some red coloured soft drinks are sour	Yes/No
Some sweet beverages are soft drinks	Yes/No
All green beverages are sweet.	Yes/No
Some soft drinks are naturally coloured	Yes/No

3. Most athletes are good runners. All good runners wear light-weight shoes.

Circle 'Yes' if the conclusion does follow. Circle 'No' if the conclusion does not follow.

No athletes wear light-weight shoes	Yes/No
Some good runners do not wear light-weight shoes	Yes/No
Some athletes wear light-weight shoes	Yes/No
Some good runners wear regular sport shoes	Yes/No
Most athletes wear light-weight shoes	Yes/No

4. All hot air balloons carry disposable ballast. Some disposable ballast is made of sandbags.

Circle 'Yes' if the conclusion does follow. Circle 'No' if the conclusion does not follow.

Some hot air balloons carry sandbags as disposable ballast	Yes/No
No hot air balloons carry water as disposable ballast	Yes/No
All hot air balloons carry sandbags as disposable ballast	Yes/No
All disposable ballast is made of sand	Yes/No
Some hot air balloons carry sandbags	Yes/No

5. All balconies are facing the seaside. Some seaside balconies have blue sunshades.

Circle 'Yes' if the conclusion does follow. Circle 'No' if the conclusion does not follow.

All sunshades are installed on the seaside	Yes/No
Some balconies have no sunshades	Yes/No
There are no sunshades on the seaside	Yes/No
All seaside balconies have blue sunshades	Yes/No
No seaside balconies have blue sunshades	Yes/No

6. Olympic triathlon and decathlon athletes are taking part in a display for the opening ceremony. All male triathlon athletes are to hold red rings and all female decathlon athletes are to hold blue rings. The rest of the triathlon and decathlon athletes will hold green rings.

Circle 'Yes' if the conclusion does follow. Circle 'No' if the conclusion does not follow.

All decathlon athletes are holding green rings.	Yes/No
Some triathlon athletes are holding red rings.	Yes/No
All female triathlon athletes are holding green rings.	Yes/No
Some decathlon athletes are holding green rings.	Yes/No
All decathlon athletes are holding green rings.	Yes/No

Logic Puzzles

7. Joshua, Michaela, Corina, Minna, and Jeffrey are 5 friends who each have one pet. Together they have two cats, two dogs and a goldfish. There are two white and two black pets. Jeffrey jogs with his black dog every morning. His wife, Michaela, is allergic to cats. Joshua helps pet-sitting Jeffrey's and Michaela's pets when needed, but not on Sundays when he refreshes his pet's water tank. This Sunday Joshua will visit Corina and Minna to see Corina's new black cat. Who has a white cat?

A. Joshua   B. Michaela   C. Corina   D. Minna

8. It is Mother's Day and five friends (Denise, Flavia, Anne, Mary, and Diane) are buying flowers for their moms, each picking her mom's favourites. They ordered five bunches: one with lilies, one with lilac and the others with roses. Each bunch is a different colour. Denise picked the orange flowers, but these were not roses. Flavia picked yellow, Mary red, and Diane purple flowers. Anne chose the white roses. Only two mothers received roses on Mother's Day and neither bunch was purple. Which of the friends are siblings?

A. Denise & Diane   B. Flavia & Anne   C. Mary & Denise   D. Flavia & Diane

9. The summer Olympic games will include football, basketball, handball, volley and gymnastics. Only two team sports have matching T-shirts and pants. Basketball players wear white short pants and orange T-shirts. Volley players do not wear blue and football players wear red matching outfits. The gymnast wears orange pants and green T-shirt. Who wears blue pants?

A. Handball team   B. Football team   C. Basketball team   D. Volley team

10. Four friends (Claudia, Brandon, Kim, James) go out for an Italian pasta dinner. They order tortellini, ravioli, penne and spaghetti, each with a different specialty sauce. Brandon ordered ravioli with cheese and Kim wanted penne. James does not like fungi or ragu sauce, but loves pesto. Claudia does not like fungi either, but ordered ragu with tortellini. Who ordered spaghetti and who likes fungi?

A. Claudia & Brandon   C. Kim & Brandon

B. Brandon & James   D. James & Kim

11. Four classmates were asked to choose their favourite music genre and sport in a personality test. Tania, James, Meera and Rob each liked a different sport and different genre of music. The music genres chosen were rock, pop, classical and rap. The sports chosen were cricket, hockey, badminton and football.

Tania's favourite sport is badminton

James favourite music genre is rap and Robert's favourite genre is rock. The person whose favourite genre is pop, their favourite sport is hockey.

Which of the following must be true?

A. James' favourite sport is cricket

B. Rob's favourite sport is football

C. The person whose favourite sport is cricket rated rap music their favourite.

D. Tania's favourite music genre is classical

Recognising Assumptions

12. Should we introduce nationwide guaranteed minimum income to reduce poverty?
    A. Yes, giving people money ensures more children will be fed better.
    B. Yes, by providing everyone with a guaranteed income higher than the poverty limit, fewer people will be impoverished.
    C. No, giving everyone money will merely cause them to lose the motivation to work and become impoverished.
    D. No, the cost of giving everyone money will bankrupt the country.

13. Should all gluten be made illegal to protect people with celiac disease from having a reaction to it?
    Yes, if gluten is illegal someone with celiac disease cannot access it and have a reaction to it.
    Yes, gluten causes weight gain if eaten in excess.
    No, people with celiac disease do not care if you eat gluten.
    No, gluten is an important ingredient in many foods.

14. Should homes only be allowed to flush their toilets twice a day to prevent causing a drought?
    A. Yes, flushing toilets accounts for most of the water consumption in the cities.
    B. Yes, people would not be at home during the day anyway and do not need to flush the toilet more than twice.
    C. No, not flushing toilets would reduce the income of water treatment service companies, reducing the availability of potable water.
    D. No, droughts are caused by climactic events that are not influenced by the flushing of toilets.

15. Should all public payphones be removed to save taxpayers money?
    A. Yes, the latest usage reports show that very few calls are placed in a fiscal year.
    B. Yes, the tax revenue due to profits from the few calls made on public phones is minimal.
    C. No, red phone booths are an iconic image and should not be removed.
    D. No, public payphones are run by private businesses at no cost to taxpayer.

16. Should the selective breeding of brachycephalic dogs (pugs, boxers, bulldogs, etc.) be banned to reduce the number of health problems these breeds are now prone to?

A. Yes, it has been demonstrated that the selective breeding of brachycephalic breeds in particular has led to an overwhelming set of debilitating health problems for these breeds.

B. Yes, on average a pug born today will suffer from airway obstruction, an inability to properly close its eyes, and infections of the skin folds on its snout.

C. No, brachycephalic breeds have become some of the highest priced and most in demand breeds of dogs due to the perceived "cuteness" of having a short snout.

D. No, responsible ownership, not responsible breeding practices, is important.

17. Should nuclear power plants be eliminated to prevent radiation leaks caused by reactor meltdowns?

A. Yes, eliminating all nuclear power plants would indeed eliminate the risk of radiation being leaked by a reactor meltdown.

B. Yes, the transport and disposal of spent fuel rods is an ongoing challenge with a high risk for radiation to be leaked.

C. No, nuclear power generation is still one of the most reliable low carbon emission power sources available and eliminating it would leave a large gap in the power supply that could only be filled by fossil fuel power plants.

D. No, research and improved engineering will increase the efficiency of nuclear power maximizing the usefulness of this source of energy.

Interpreting Information

18. The survival results of a drug trial comparing two different drugs to a placebo are presented below. Decide whether the following conclusions follow:

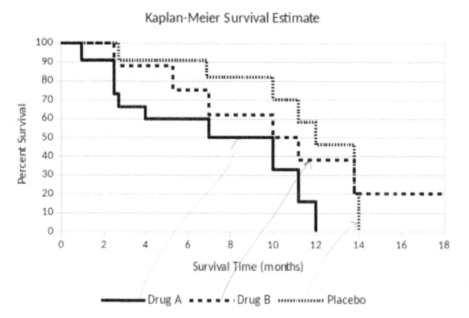

Kaplan-Meier Survival Estimate

—— Drug A - - - - Drug B ·············· Placebo

A. Patients prescribed Drug A had better survival compared to those prescribed Drug B.　Yes/No

B. Median survival time, the time it took for 50% of the patients in a particular treatment group to die, was longest in the group receiving Drug B.　Yes/No

C. After 13 months most of the patients had died.　Yes/No

D. For most of the study the placebo group had the highest % of patients alive.　Yes/No

19. The table below shows the breakdown of two types of hospital admissions and their associated costs over 5 years. Decide whether the following conclusions follow:

Numbers (millions)	2012	2013	2014	2015	2016
Emergency Admissions	4.90	5.39	5.93	6.52	7.17
In-patient Admissions	9.70	12.13	15.16	18.95	23.68
Overall Cost	10,690.0	13,068.5	16,012.2	19,659.5	24,183.1

A. There were more in-patient admissions than emergency room admissions between 2012 than ₂₀₁₆　Yes/No

B. The average rate of increase in emergency room admissions over 5 years was greater than the rate of increase in in-patient admissions for the same period.　Yes/No

C. There were consistently only twice as many in-patient admissions as emergency room admissions.   Yes/No

D. The number of emergency room admissions increased by about 10% each year.   Yes/No

20. Sports fans from various countries were asked whether they prefer to watch football or cricket, the poll results are graphed below. The size of the bubble corresponds to the percentage of that nationality which preferred the given sport. Each bubble is also centred on that same percentage relative to the y-axis. Decide whether the following conclusions follow:

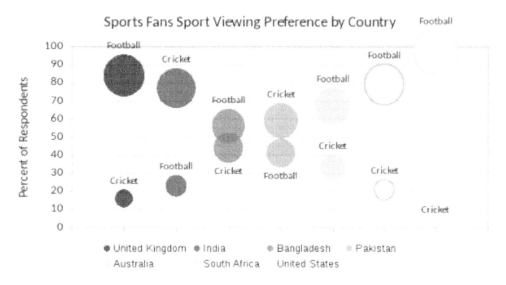

A. Sports fans from the United States dislike cricket the most.   Yes/No

B. Bangladesh is the closest to an even split between preference for watching football and preference for watching cricket.   Yes/No

C. Australia is the closest to having exactly twice as many sports fans that prefer watching football to cricket.   Yes/No

D. The United Kingdom has the highest proportion of sports fans that would prefer to watch football.   Yes/No

21. The graph below shows the number of beats per minute (BPM) for four people's top 5 favourite songs, Song 1 is their favourite, song 5 is their 5th favourite. Decide whether the following conclusions follow:

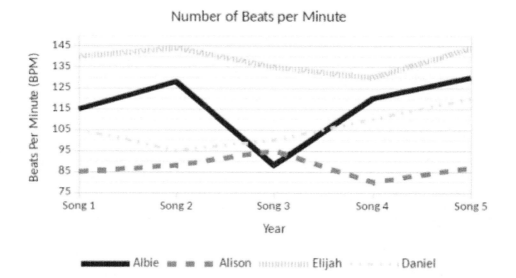

A. Alison generally favours songs with fewer BPM than the other three.   Yes/No

B. Elijah's favourite song has more BPM than all the other people's favourite song.   Yes/No

C. Albie's top five favourite songs are spread across a wider range of speeds than the other people's.   Yes/No

D. Women usually like fewer BPM in their music than men.   Yes/No

22. The pie charts show the percentage of new cars sold with each of the corresponding colours for two major car manufacturers. Land Rover on the Left and Jaguar on the right. Decide whether the following conclusions follow:

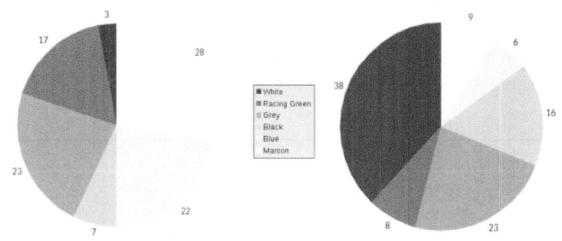

A. Both manufacturers sell more white cars than any other individual colour.   Yes/No

B. Half of all jaguars sold are either blue or maroon.   Yes/No

C. Both manufacturers sell the same percentage of grey cars.   Yes/No

D. The most common colour choice for any one manufacturer is white.   Yes/No

23. The chart below shows the total monthly sales of 3 restaurant branches in a city.

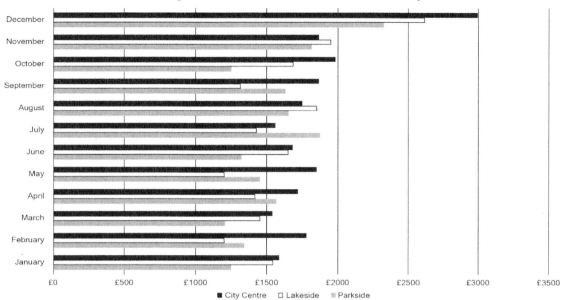

Chart showing sales at 3 restaurant branches for year 2015

A. In the month of March, the branch which generated the lowest amount of sale was the Lakeside branch. Yes/No

B. The Parkside branch generated more sale than the Lakeside branch in July Yes/No

C. The highest total amount of sale for all three branches was generated in the month of January. Yes/No

D. The only months which saw the City Centre branch's sales fall lower than the preceding month were March and July. Yes/No

Probability

24. In order to win a large prize at a carnival Amelia must guess what 4-digit number a random number generator will create. Amelia knows the first digit is always a 1, the second digit can only be either 7 or 0, the third digit can only be a 1, 3, or 9, while the fourth digit can be any number. Amelia thinks she has at least a 1 in 100 chance. Is Amelia correct in thinking she has at least a 1% chance of winning?

A. Yes, her chance of winning is 1/14

B. Yes, her chance of winning is 1/60

C. No, her chance of winning is 1/60

D. No, her chance of winning is 1/14

25. Jacob is playing a card game with a standard deck of 52 cards (13 cards of each suit). He is the first to draw a card and hopes it will be either an Ace or a black card. Is the chance for Jacob to draw either and Ace or a black card greater than 1/2?

A. Yes, the chance to draw an Ace or black card is 13/26

B. Yes, the chance to draw an Ace or black card is 7/13

C. No, the chance to draw an Ace or black card is 7/13

D. No, the chance to draw an Ace or black card is 13/26

26. Oliver is in line to win one of three new tablets. Contestants need to draw one of 3 red chips in a jar to win. At the start of the contest there were 44 yellow chips 27 green chips and 25 blue chips. So far 39 people have drawn a chip and 1 tablet has been won. Are Oliver's chances of winning now better than if he had drawn first?

A. Yes, his probability was 1/33 but is now 1/30

B. Yes, his probability was 1/30 but is now 1/39

C. No, his probability was 1/30 but is now 1/39

D. No, his probability was 1/30 but is now 1/30

27. Aiden is in line at a carnival to spin a prize wheel. The wheel has 12 equally sized sectors and each sector corresponds to a prize. 5 of the sectors correspond to small prizes, 2 sectors correspond to medium prizes, 1 sector corresponds to a large prize, 1 sector is the grand prize, and 3 sectors correspond to winning no prize. So far Aiden has seen 7 children take a turn before him. 3 of them won small prizes, 3 won no prize, and 1 won a large prize. Does Aiden have a higher probability of winning the grand prize now than if he had spun first?

A. Yes, Aiden now has a chance of 1/5

B. Yes, Aiden now has a chance of 1/12

C. No, Aiden now has a chance of 1/12

D. No, Aiden now has a chance of 1/5

28. Abigail cannot decide whether she wants to have chicken, salmon, pork, or turkey. She decides to flip a coin if she gets 2 heads in a row she will have chicken, if she gets a heads and then a tails she will have salmon, if she gets tails and then heads she will have pork, and finally if she flips 2 tails she will have turkey. Her first flip was tails. Has the chance that Abigail will have turkey doubled?

A. Yes, her chance was 1/4 and is now 0/4

B. Yes, her chance was 1/4 and is now 1/2

C. No, her chance was 1/4 and is now 1/2

D. No, her chance was 1/4 and is now 0/4

Venn Diagrams

29. An apartment building has 19 flats and two garages, one red and one blue, allowing 1 parking spot per flat. The red garage is smaller than half of the blue garage. If we move all the cars from the red garage into the blue garage, the remainder space in the half of the garage could fit 2 cars. How many cars may fit in the blue garage?

A. 9   B. 12   C. 14   D. 19

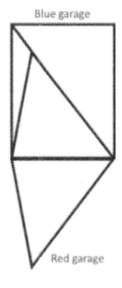

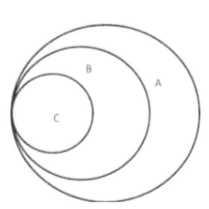

30. The barman prepared 25 cocktails decorated with lemons. Of these, 1 in 5 also had fresh mint. For each drink with fresh mint he prepared another 2 without mint. All other drinks had one lemon and one cherry per cocktail. How many cherries did he need for the order?

A. 15   C. 5

B. 10   D. 25

31. Today's fashion show presents a total of 7 dresses, 8 hats, and 10 scarfs. Some are matching colours, while some have various prints. They introduce a matching red set including dress, hat and scarf. There are 2 pairs of black hats and dresses, 2 of hats and scarfs that are blue and more than one white scarf and dress set. The show presents two floral dresses. How many multicolour hats and scarfs are to be introduced during the show?

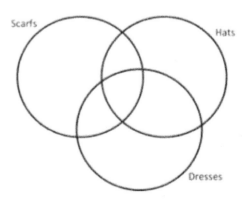

A. 3&5   B. 5&3   C. 3&2   D. 2&3

32. A fragrance company have fragrances made up of the ingredients in the key below. Some fragrances only have one ingredient whereas others are a mixture of ingredients.

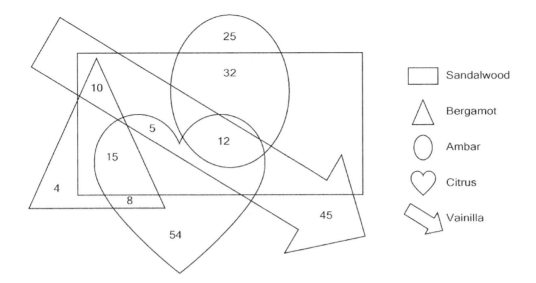

Based on the diagram, how many fragrances consisted of a mixture of bergamot, citrus, and sandalwood?

A. 15

B. 10

C. 12

D. 5

Solutions

Syllogisms

Question 1

Conclusion 1 - No - this conclusion makes an assumption that all individuals with dark skin are vitamin D deficient which directly contradicts the second premise that only "some individuals with dark skin are vitamin D deficient".

Conclusion 2 - No - The individuals with dark skin who are vitamin D deficient may not be Europeans of African descent, for example Africans or Indians instead.

Conclusion 3 - No - the assumption is not supported by the premises

Conclusion 4- No - See Conclusion 2.

Conclusion 5 - No - this directly contradicts the first premise that "All Europeans of African descent have dark skin"

Question 2

Conclusion 1 - Yes - the second premise tells us that sweet beverages are artificially coloured, thus if all soft drinks are sweet it is reasonable to assume that all will also be artificially coloured.

Conclusion 2 - No - this directly contradicts the first premise that all soft drinks are sweet.

Conclusion 3 - Yes - the first premise states that all soft drinks are sweet, then it is correct to assume that some of the beverages that are sweet are also soft drinks.

Conclusion 4 - No - the assumption is not supported by the premises.

Conclusion 5 - No - this contradicts both premises. If all soft drinks are sweet and sweet beverages are artificially coloured, then the correct assumption is that all soft drinks are artificially coloured, therefore some soft drinks cannot be naturally coloured.

Question 3

Conclusion 1 - No - this conclusion contradicts the first premise as it assumes that no athletes are good runners.

Conclusion 2 - No - this conclusion directly contradicts the second premise stating that all good runners wear light-weight shoes.

Conclusion 3 - Yes - the first premise states that most athletes are good runners and the second premise tells us that all good runners wear light-weight shoes, therefore there are some athletes that wear light-weight shoes.

Conclusion 4 - No - this conclusion directly contradicts the second premise stating that all good runners wear light-weight shoes.

Conclusion 5 - Yes - the first premise states that most athletes are good runners and the second premise tells us that all good runners wear light-weight shoes, therefore it is reasonable to assume that most athletes wear light-weight shoes.

Question 4

Conclusion 1 – Yes – since all hot air balloons carry disposable ballast and some ballast is made of sand, it is reasonable to assume that some balloons carry sand disposable ballast.

Conclusion 2 – No – the assumption is not supported by the premises.

Conclusion 3 – No – this assumption contradicts the second premise. Only some disposable ballast is made of sandbags, thus some other may be made of something else. Hence it is incorrect to assume that all hot air balloons carry sandbags as disposable ballast.

Conclusion 4 – No – this assumption directly contradicts the second premise, that some disposable ballast is made of sandbags.

Conclusion 5 – Yes – we know that all hot air balloons carry disposable ballast and some disposable ballast is made of sand. Thus, we can correctly assume that some hot air balloons may carry sand.

Question 5

Conclusion 1 – No – the assumption is not supported by the premises.

Conclusion 2 – No – this cannot be determined given these premises. Although it is stated some sun shades are blue, we can't assume some balconies have no sun shades from just the second statement.

Conclusion 3 – No – this assumption contradicts the second premise, that some sea side balconies have blue sun shades.

Conclusion 4 – No – this assumption directly contradicts the second premise, that only some sea side balconies have blue sun shades.

Conclusion 5 – No – this assumption contradicts the second premise

Question 6

Read the information carefully, identifying the variables involved and what the question is asking you to evaluate. We are being asked to identify which conclusions follow based on the information we are provided with. Break down the information we are given:

Triathlon and decathlon athletes are present

Male triathlon = red rings

Female decathlon = blue rings

Remainder = green rings

Conclusion 1 – No – only male decathlon athletes will be holding green rings; the female decathlon athletes are holding blue rings.

Conclusion 2 – Yes – the male triathlon athletes are holding red rings.

Conclusion 3 – Yes – we are told male triathlon athletes are holding red rings and the rest of the triathlon athletes are holding green rings. This means all female athletes must be holding green rings.

Conclusion 4 – Yes – we're told female decathlon-ers hold blue rings, the rest of the decathlon.

Logic Puzzles

Question 7

Everyone has a pet. Jeffrey and Michaela have two pets of which one is a black dog, Michaela is allergic to cats. It is not sure what kind of pet Joshua has, but we know that he will refresh his pet's water tank on Sunday's. Thus, Joshua has the goldfish and Michaela has the second dog. Corina has a new black cat, so Jeffrey and Corina have the two black pets. Michaela's dog must be white. Since Minna does not have a pet, she must be the second cat owner which is also the second white pet.

Question 8

We notice there are 3 bunches of roses. Since all friends picked mom's favoured flowers and two are siblings, then we can conclude that two of the three friends buying roses are siblings. Denise picked the orange flowers, but these were not roses. Therefore, we can conclude that Denise is not one of the siblings, hence the answers "Denise and Diane" and "Mary and Denise" must be incorrect. Diane bought purple flowers, but we know that neither mom received purple flowers. Thus, Diane did not offer roses to her mom which indicates that she is not one of the siblings either, leaving "Flavia and Anne" as the only correct option

Question 9

We know that only two teams wear matching outfits and the football team wears matching red outfits, we know that the football players do not wear blue. Basketball team is an incorrect answer (since they wear white/orange). The puzzle specifically states that the volley players do not wear blue. Therefore, the handball team is the correct answer.

Question 10

Since Brandon ordered ravioli, Claudia tortellini and Kim penne, we can assume that James ordered spaghetti. Brandon got the cheese sauce, Claudia ordered ragu and James pesto. Thus, Kim is the only that could have ordered fungi sauce and "James & Kim" is correct.

Question 11

Read the question carefully and register the number of individuals and variables involved. Create a table: You may be pushed for time but quickly jot the information that is certain down into a table to begin eliminating answer options.

Name	Sport	Music
Tania	Badminton	
James		Rap
Meera	Hockey	Pop
Rob	Sport	Rock

In these questions, some answers could potentially be true but the questions asks which statement MUST be true taking into account all the information. There is only one unknown in terms of music genre but two unknowns in terms of favourite sport. D is the only option which must be true.

Recognising Assumptions

Question 12

B. is the strongest argument because it directly relates the action with the effect; providing everyone with enough money to not live in poverty will reduce the number of individuals considered impoverished.

A. while more children may receive better nutrition, this is neither the aim of providing guaranteed income, nor supported by provided evidence.

C. while this argument discusses both the action, giving money, and the effect, the state of poverty, it relies on the assumption that people will lose motivation to remain un-impoverished.

D. this argument discusses the action but not the effect and, thus, is not the strongest argument.

Question 13

A. addresses both components of the aim of the question, specifically making gluten illegal will prevent people with celiac disease from having reactions to gluten.

B. does not address the aim of the question at all.

C. does not address the aim of the question, regardless of whether someone with celiac disease cares if others consume it, the aim is whether or not making it illegal will prevent reactions to gluten.

D. does not address the aim of the question.

Question 14

D. is the strongest argument because it addresses both components of the aim of the question.

A. does not draw any link between the water consumed by toilets and the causes of droughts.

B. both assumes that people will have no need to flush their home toilets more than twice and fails to address the effect. C. does not address the effect of the question.

Question 15

D. is the best argument because it addresses both the action and effect.

A. points out that few calls are made but this does not address the effect of saving money.

B. actually suggests that there is some small tax revenue and that eliminating them would cost taxpayers.

C. does not address either the action or the effect.

Question 16

A. is the strongest argument because it provides evidence of how the action is directly related to the effect in the aim of the question.

B. addresses the effect in question but provides no evidence that the proposed action will produce the desired effect.

C. does not address either the action or the effect in question.

D. does not address the action or effect in question and rather tries to deflect the aim of the question.

Question 17

A. directly addresses both the action and the effect of the aim.

B. does not address the action or the specific effect of reactor meltdown. Neither B nor

C. address the specific aims of the question.

Interpreting Information

Question 18

Conclusion 1 - No - Drug A had the lowest percent of patients alive at any given time after the first month of the study and, therefore, had poorer survival than Drug B.

Conclusion 2 - No - the placebo group had the longest median survival time (>12 months) while the median survival time for Drug A was about 7 months and was 10 months for Drug B.

Conclusion 3 - Yes - by 13 months all of the patients treated with Drug A had died and over 50% of those in the remaining groups had also died meaning that over half of all patients had died.

Conclusion 4 - Yes - for over 10 months of the 18 months studied the placebo group had highest percentage of patients alive.

Question 19

Conclusion 1 - Yes - one can easily see that there were more in-patient admissions for every year on record, therefore, there must have been more in-patient admissions. Alternatively, 4.9+5.39+5.93+6.52+7.17=29.91, while 9.7+12.13+15.16+18.95+23.68=79.62.

Conclusion 2 - No - one can see that the number of emergency room visits per year in 2016 did not double as compared to 2012 while the number of in-patient admissions per year more than doubled in the same period. Therefore, the annual rate of increase in admissions must be greater for the in-patient admissions

Conclusion 3 - No - with the exception of 2012 there were more than twice as many in-patient admissions as emergency room admissions with more than triple as many in-patient admissions as emergency room admissions in 2016.

Conclusion 4 -Yes - one can simply add 10% to each year and see that it equals almost exactly the next year's emergency room admissions. 4.9 + (0.1 x 4.9) = 5.39, 5.39 + (0.1 x 5.39) = 5.929, which is about 5.93. 5.93 + (0.1 x 5.93) = 6.523, which is about 6.52. 6.52 + (0.1 x 6.52) = 7.172, which is about 7.17. Therefore, emergency room admissions did increase by about 10% each year.

Question 20

Conclusion 1 - No - while the Unites States had the fewest respondents that prefer was cricket, a preference for watching football does not imply a dislike of cricket.

Conclusion 2 - Yes - the two groups in Bangladesh exhibit the most amount of overlap. A perfectly even split would be 50% in each group resulting in perfectly overlapped bubbles.

Conclusion 3 - Yes - an exact 1 to 2 split of the 100% of Australian respondents would be 33.33% preferring cricket and 66.67% preferring football. Australian respondents are indeed the closest to achieving this.

Conclusion 4 - No - the proportion, or percentage, of sports fans from the United Kingdom that would prefer to watch football is roughly 84 – 85% while the proportion of United States sports fans, the only nation to exceed the United Kingdom in preference for watching football, that prefer watching football is >95%.

Question 21

Conclusion 1 - Yes - the slowest song pick of all is Alison's and each of her other songs are slower than their matched comparators with the exception of Albie's song 3 pick.

Conclusion 2 - Yes - not only does Elijah's favourite song, Song 1, have more BPM than everyone else's favourite song, all of his 5 favourite songs have more BPM than all the five choices of everyone else.

Conclusion 3 - Yes - the fastest song in Albie's 5 favourites is Song 5 at 130 BPM while the slowest is Song 3 at about 83 BPM meaning Albie's favourite songs are spread across a range of almost 50 BPM which is clearly greater than all the others.

Conclusion 4 -No - there is no information presented on BPM preferences by sex and thus this conclusion cannot be draw.

Question 22

Conclusion 1 - No - only Land Rover sells more white cars than any other colour.

Conclusion 2 -Yes - 28% of Jaguars sold are maroon and 22% are blue, 28% + 22% = 50%.

Conclusion 3 - Yes - grey cars represent 23% percent of new car sales for both manufacturers.

Conclusion 4 - Yes - 38% of new Land Rovers sold are white. 38% is the highest percentage of new cars for any one manufacturer to be the same colour.

Question 23

Eyeball the data and what information is being represented. We have been given the monthly sales of different restaurant branches in a city. The sales are given in pounds (£).

Evaluate each statement in turn. Eyeball the extreme values and familiarise yourself with the key and which colour represents which restaurant.

Conclusion 1 -No- because the branch with the lowest sales in March was in fact, the Parkside branch.

Conclusion 2 -Yes- because the Parkside branch generated roughly £1,800 in July compared to Lakeside branch which generated less than £1,500.

Conclusion 3 -No- because the month which saw the highest amount of sales for all three branches was December. (Be careful to read the axis carefully. The month at the top is December)

Conclusion 4 -No- because there was a fall in sales occurred at the City Centre branch In March, June and July.

Probability

Question 24

The first digit is always a 1 so Amelia has a 1/1 chance of guessing the first digit, the second digit can only be 1 of 2 options, so Amelia has a 1/2 chance of guessing the second digit, the third digit is 1 of 3 options and the last digit is 1 of 10 options. Therefore, Amelia's chance of guessing all for digits correctly is 1/1x1/2x1/3x1/10=1/60 and 1/60 is greater than 1/100 or 1% so Amelia indeed has at least a 1/100 chance.

Question 25

First, the number of possible cards out of 52 that will satisfy Jacob's hope is 28. There are 4 Aces and 26 black cards in a deck of cards. Two of the Aces are also black, therefore, the total number of cards in the deck that would either be an Ace or black are 26+2=28. Thus, Jacobs chances of drawing one of these cards is 28/52=7/13 and 7/13 is greater than 1/2.

Question 26

It might be helpful to write down on a sticky note and stick it near your desk whilst you're doing UCAT practice with the setup of a standard deck of cards. As in how many of everything. There can be a few questions to do with cards and you don't want to miss out on valuable marks.

A) Had Oliver drawn first his chances of winning, would have been 3 out of the total number of chips. So, 3 red + 44 yellow + 27 green + 25 blue = 99 total chips, therefore, his original chance would have been 3/99 = 1/33. However, currently there are 39 less total chips and 1 less winning red chip. So, 2 red out of 99 - 39 = 2/60, therefore, his current chance is 1/30.

Question 27

C) Aiden's chance of winning the grand prize has not changed and, therefore, cannot be higher. Every time the wheel is spun there is the same chance of winning the grand prize because previous outcomes do not affect the current spin. There were originally 12 sectors that could be landed on, 1 of which was the grand prize. So, the chance of winning was 1/12, since the number of sectors and the corresponding prizes has not changed, Aiden still has a 1/12 chance of winning the grand prize.

B) To begin, each flip had a 1/2 chance to be either side, so any one meat choice had a probability of being selected of 1/2 x 1/2 = 1/4 before Abigail started flipping a coin. Since the result of the first flip is now know the subsequent flip has a 1/2 chance to be the needed side. Importantly, turkey is possible to be selected since the first flip result was tails which eliminated chicken and salmon as options. But is 1/2 double 1/4: (1/2) / (1/4) = (1/2) / (1/2 x 1/2) = 2. So, yes, Abigail's chance of having turkey has doubled.

Venn Diagrams

Blue garage

Question 29

There are 19 total parking spots between the two garages of the building. We know that the number of parking spots in the red garage plus 2 equals half of the number of parking spots in the blue garage. If we subtract 2 from 19, then 17 is the number of parking spots in half of the blue garage plus twice the number of parking spots in the red garage. If we subtract 2 from 17, then 15 will represent 3 times the number of parking spots in the red garage. Thus, the red garage has 5 parking spots and the blue garage has (5+2) X 2 = 14 parking spots.

Question 30

For a total of 25 cocktails, 1 in 5 indicates that 5 cocktail drinks had lemon and fresh mint. 5x2=10 with lemon without fresh mint. Lemon and cherry cocktails were 25-5-10= 10. Therefore, the correct answer is "10 cherries".

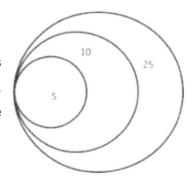

Question 31

The total number of pieces presented: 7+8+10=25. There are 2 black hats, 2 blue hats and 1 red hat, thus 8-2-2-1=3 multicoloured hats. There are 2 black dresses, 2 floral dresses and 1 red dress, thus 7-2-2-1=2 white dresses (more than one scarf and dress set). Hence, the show introduces 2 white scarfs, 2 black scarfs, 1 red scarf and the rest are multicoloured. 10-2-2-1=5 multicoloured scarfs. The answer "3&5" is correct.

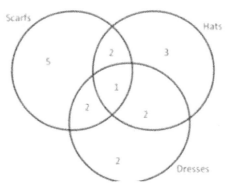

Question 32

Reading the question, identify what information the question is asking us to determine. We have been given data relating to the readership of different magazines and then presented with a choice Venn diagrams. The question is asking us to identify which Venn diagram reflects the data collected.

Picture the information, using key pieces of information we can begin to form parts of the Venn diagram and the numbers which should be found in unique parts. For example, we know 2 people read all three magazines so 2 should be found in the centre-most overlap.

Discard and Decide: Using key data we can begin to eliminate options which are incorrect and move closer to the correct answer. In this question, we can't rule out any options based on those that read all three magazines since 2 is found in every answer option's centremost overlap. However, we can eliminate D based on the fact 5 people read no magazines, this is represented by the number outside the diagram. D has 4 placed outside the diagram and is therefore incorrect. We know the total number of students asked was 50, so all the numbers in the diagram should total this value. This rules out C. Now identify which circle represents which magazine. 30 read Science Report monthly, so look for a circle where all the values add up to 30. This is both A and B. 15 read Today's Experiment. Only answer option B has a circle (bottom) which totals this value and we can therefore discard A and select B as our correct answer.

Quantitative Reasoning

What is 'Quantitative Reasoning'?

UCAT examiners are quick to point out that the Quantitative Reasoning section of the exam is more focused on testing problem solving skills than mathematical ability alone. For the most part, we think that this is true; the questions themselves often give a table, graph or some other form of diagram with an attached scenario, and it's up to you to use maths to interpret this data and answer the problem.

However, there's no escaping from the fact that you are going to be expected to be familiar with maths at a GCSE level and will have to know and be able to use various formulae and mathematical concepts. It should be noted that the UCAT does not examine the entire GCSE maths syllabus, but rather questions are focused in certain areas.

Why do we have to do QR?

Possessing a solid foundation in basic maths is crucial throughout medical school, and also throughout your career as a doctor or dentist. Doctors deal with numbers every day and being able to interpret and analyse data quickly and accurately is essential.

You'll most likely meet medical statistics upon starting university, and not long after, you'll be calculating drug dosages and analysing graphs. The level of mathematical knowledge required of a doctor isn't very high - rather, a firm understanding of basic maths, and knowing how to apply it to simple problems is what counts. The QR section reflects this, so brushing up on your maths skills will put you in good stead for the future.

Here's a simple example of a problem you'll come across at medical school:

An obese man, weighing 112 kg, is hypotensive and has low cardiac output. His cardiologist decides to start a dopamine drip starting at 20 mcg/kg/min. How many milligrams would this patient receive in 1 hr?

Firstly, the doctor (or nurse) must convert micrograms (mcg) to milligrams (mg):

$$\frac{1}{0.001} = \frac{20}{x}$$

By cross-multiplication and division, we can work out 20 mcg = 0.02 mg.

This patient weights 112 kg, therefore he would receive: 0.02 x 112 kg = 2.24 mg/min.

In 60 minutes, this patient will receive: 2.24 x 60 = 134.4 mg/hour.

This is a simple illustration of using a conversion factor, and also of ratios/proportions. You'll come across these basic calculations on the hospital ward, and most likely under pressure and without much time.

Numbers for this section

- **Time**

  26 minutes total = 1 minute for instructions + 25 minutes for questions

- **Questions**

  36 questions total

  9 sets (4 questions each)

You have 25 minutes to do 36 questions, as well as 1 minute to carefully read over the instructions. This means that you only have 41.5 seconds to answer each question, assuming of course that you spend the same amount of time on each problem (in reality, you'll find some easy questions can be answered in a matter of seconds whilst others will take significantly longer). As with all sections of the UCAT, efficient time management is crucial, and so it is very important to enter the exam with a set strategy and to stick to it.

Strategy

Skim, flag and review

It is no secret that not all QR questions were made equal; some will be very easy and will take only a few seconds to answer, whilst others may take significantly longer. It is therefore essential to prioritise the easier questions throughout the exam. The best way to do this is to employ the skim, flag and review technique.

- *Skim* - Skim through the question and try to pick out the relevant data or information that will be required. Mentally categorise the question difficulty as easy, medium or hard.

- *Flag* - If you have decided that the question is potentially difficult and will take considerable time to answer, guess an answer and flag it for review at the end. There is no negative marking within QR and so do not be afraid to guess the incorrect answer. It is better to put something down than to leave it blank.

- *Review* - If you have time at the end you can return to the more difficult questions that you have only guessed the answer for and attempt to work them out.

It is important to be conscious of time throughout the exam; you should aim to finish each set in roughly 2 minutes or less to make good time. Spending too long on one question can result in later questions being missed that are considerably easier. We recommend that at the beginning of the 5th set of questions, you should have roughly 16 minutes remaining; if you are behind a set or more, you should start to flag more questions to ensure you can answer all of those that are easier. If you are only slightly behind, there is less urgency to flag; the aim of the game is not to answer every single question, it's to answer as many questions correctly in the allotted time. If you are ahead of schedule, there is less urgency to flag questions, although be aware that you might spend longer than you think on a question yet to come.

To put it simply - by the halfway mark, if you're:

- *Behind by a set or more* - it's important you start flagging and moving on from the harder questions. Through practice, you'll begin to be more aware of the more time-consuming questions - flag these and move on, otherwise you'll be missing out on easy marks.

- *Slightly behind* - still consider flagging, guessing, and skipping the hard questions. Remember, the aim of the game isn't to finish every single question - it's to get as many questions right as possible in the time allotted.

- *On target or faster* - you should be on track to finish every question as long as you don't get held back on a complex question. If a question looks like it's going to require more than 30 seconds, the safest strategy is to flag it, guess and move on.

Mental Arithmetic

Whilst you will be provided with an on-screen calculator in the exam, typing numbers into it will use precious time that could be spent answering questions. It is a bad habit to rely on the calculator for every question regardless of how simple it is. Being able to mentally solve simple maths problems will give a huge advantage when taking this exam and so it is important to solve problems in your head as often as is possible.

Lots of this will be super straightforward to many of you - or you'll have your own shortcuts which you've developed over time. But many students have found these methods helpful - so we keep them here to help!

Mental Addition and Subtraction

- The key to quicker mental calculation is to simplify.
- Do this by breaking a calculation up into bits.

Addition Examples:

- 2-digit e.g. 37+42 = 37 + 40 + 2 = 77 + = 79
- 3-digit e.g. 438 + 327 = 438 + 300+20+7 = 738 + 20 + 7 = 758 + 7 = 765
- Rounding e.g. 448 + 298 = 450 - 2 + 300 - 2 = 750 - 2 - 2 = 746

Subtraction Examples:

- 2-digit e.g. 57-34 = 57 - 30 - 4 = 27 - 4 = 23
- 3-digit e.g. 847 - 234 = 847 - 200 - 30 - 4 = 647 - 30 - 4 = 617 - 4 = 613
- Rounding e.g. 748 - 298 = 750 - 2 - 300 + 2 = 450

Mental Multiplication

- Again, simplification makes harder calculations easier to handle, and also reduces the temptation of using a calculator.
- As long as you know your times tables up to 10, you'll be able to implement the below methods easily and hopefully see a substantial increase in calculating sums mentally.

Examples:

- Multiplying by 11, e.g. 25 x 11
  - Add the two digits of the number being multiplied ('7')
  - Put the answer between the two digits of the number being multiplied (2 7 5)
- 2-by-1, e.g. 43 x 6
  - Separate: (40+3) x 6
  - Multiply separately: 40x6=240, 3x6=18
  - Add together: 240+18=258

- Rounding, e.g. 59 x 7
  - Separate: (60-1) x 7
  - Multiply separately: 60x7=420, -1x7=-7
  - Add together: 420-7=413
- 3-by-1, e.g. 853 x 8
  - Separate: (800+50+3)x8
  - Multiply separately: 800x8=6400, 50x8=400, 3x8=24
  - Add together: 6,400+400+24=6,824
- 2-by-2 (harder and requires a bit more practice) e.g. 37 x 82
  - Separate: (30+7) x 80 = 2400 + 560 = 2960
  - (30+7) x 2 = 60 + 14 = 74
  - Add together: 3034
- Subtraction method (easier if number ends in 9 or 8), e.g. 79 x 47
  - Round-up: 80 x (40+7) = 3200 + 560 = 3760
  - Subtract 1 lot of 47 = 3760 - 47 = 3,713

Squaring

- Anything that ends in a 5, e.g 15
  - Take the first digit(s) before the 5 and add 1 (='2' in this case)
  - Multiply the answer with the digit(s) before 5 (=2 x 1 = 2)
  - Chuck on 25 on the end (=225)
- Any 2-digit number, e.g. 14
  - Take any 2-digit number and add or subtract the necessary amount to attain a round number (i.e. 10), do the opposite addition/subtraction (if you subtracted 4 from 14 to get 10, add on 4 to get 18)
  - Multiply the results (18 x 10)
  - Add on the squared second digit (180 + 4^2 = 196)

Estimation

Another great way to save time in the exam is to estimate answers (where appropriate) rather than using a calculator. Estimation is appropriate where the range of possible answers given is wide, so that the inaccuracy caused by your estimation will not give the incorrect answer.

For example, imagine that we are told that one brick weighs 1.15 kg. We are then asked to calculate the weight of a stack of 5 bricks. We can round 1.15kg to either 1.2kg or, even better, to 1kg which will allow us to find an approximate answer much faster. Of course, our answer will be slightly inaccurate and so it will only be appropriate where the range of possible answers is large.

Imagine that the possible answers are:

A. 1.15 kg   B. 5.75 kg   C. 11.50 kg   D. 17.25 kg   E. 23.00 kg

 The range of these five possible answers above is large and so the estimation method, giving us an answer of 5kg, clearly shows that the answer must be (B).

An example of a range of answers that is too narrow would be:

A. 5.70 kg   B. 5.75 kg   C. 5.80 kg   D. 5.85 kg   E. 5.90 kg

Here the answers are so close to one another, the estimation would be too imprecise to give the correct answer.

After reading a question, you will have to judge whether or not it is appropriate to make an estimate. Generally, lots of the questions can be answered using this method.

Preparation

If there were no time limit, most students would be able to answer all of the QR questions in the UCAT correctly. The real skill is being able to work well under time pressure, which requires the application of basic maths quickly and accurately; you should enter the exam prepared and be able to answer questions as though they are second nature. The best way to do this is to prepare by answering as many practice questions as possible. There will often be common patterns or themes used in multiple questions. Being able to spot these based on practice questions you have completed will give you a great advantage over those who cannot.

Maths Tutorials

QR tests how well you can apply basic maths to a wide range of problems. Only a limited amount of content comes up, and you certainly won't be asked to do things such as integration or trigonometry. It's important to become familiar with the different topics tested, and the question categories you'll need to tackle - this will help you react faster on test-day. The aim is to be familiar enough with the categories so that you can anticipate the questions that will come up.

Commonly tested categories:

1. Speed, Distance, Time
2. Percentages
3. Ratios & Proportions
4. Conversions
5. Probability
6. Tables & Diagrams
7. Geometry

Ensure you brush up on your basic maths before attempting any questions - go through the 'Maths' section coming up in this section, and make sure you know it back to front.

Hints and Tips

- Prioritize working on your weakest areas first; if there is a particular type of question that you know that you are particularly weak on, begin your preparation there and don't move on until you are confident in your ability to answer those questions.

- Don't necessarily check the time after every single question; this can be detrimental because it can make the psychological effects of the time pressure a lot worse. It is important to stay calm and collected to avoid making mistakes. At the same time, it is very easy to lose track of time. Perhaps check every couple of sets to ensure that you are on track. Remember to adjust your strategy accordingly depending on how far ahead or behind you are!

- You will have access to a whiteboard to use. Some questions might have multiple parts to them; use the whiteboard to keep track of any relevant information.

- When you get a question wrong in one of the practice exams, look specifically at why you got it wrong. Use the practice exams to identify areas of weakness that you need to improve upon. If you do not review any incorrect questions then you are more likely to make the same mistake in future questions, and, ultimately, the real exam.

- Aim to keep your whiteboard organized: clearly mark each question, and make sure previous working is clearly sectioned off (students can often look at the wrong part of a messy whiteboard during a question).

1. Speed, Distance & Time

A reoccurring theme within the quantitative reasoning section is questions that require calculations of speed, distance and time. Speed, distance and time are all linked by one formula which can be rearranged so that if you know two out of three of parts, you can always calculate the third. The key to this section is to learn the formula in all three of its iterations; being able to quickly recall the correct formula needed will save a great deal of time in the exam and will make it much easier to perform mental arithmetic where it is possible.

Basic Strategy

The key formula that underpins speed, distance and time questions is as follows:

$$\text{Speed} = \frac{\text{Distance}}{\text{Time}}$$

$$\text{Distance} = \text{Speed} \times \text{Time}$$

$$\text{Time} = \frac{\text{Distance}}{\text{Speed}}$$

Using this formula, if we are given a value for how far something has travelled (distance), and the time in which it spent travelling (time), we are able to calculate how fast it is travelling (speed).

This formula can be rearranged so that we can work out distance if we are given information on speed and time, or time if we are given distance and speed. The re-arranged formula will look something like this:

Another handy way of memorising this formula is to place each letter (S = speed, D = distance and T = time) in a triangle:

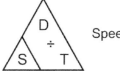 $\text{Speed} = \dfrac{\text{Distance}}{\text{Time}}$

Too quickly, work out speed, just cover up S and you are left with D/T.

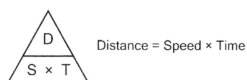 $\text{Distance} = \text{Speed} \times \text{Time}$

You can do the same with time and distance.

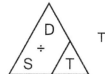 $\text{Time} = \dfrac{\text{Distance}}{\text{Speed}}$

Cover up the one you want and divide or multiply accordingly.

Advanced Techniques: Conversion of units

It should be noted here that the topic of conversion of units is covered in its own tutorial in *Conversion of units*. However, units play an especially important role when it comes to calculating speed, distance and time and so it is useful to mention them here as well.

The majority of questions will probably use the same units throughout:

Imagine that you are told that Barry cycled 60 meters in 120 seconds.

Using our formula, we can say that Barry travelled at a speed of 60/120, or 0.5, meters per second.

Notice that all of the units remain constant throughout; we are using meters as a measure of distance, seconds as a measure of time and meters per second as a measure of speed.

This is all great stuff, but things get trickier when the units are not constant throughout the question:

Let's say that we are told that Barry travelled 60 meters in 2 minutes, and that the possible answers to the question are all in meters per second (not meters per minute!).

We have to convert the units from minutes into seconds to give the correct answer.

There are 60 seconds in a minute and so simply multiply the number of minutes we have been given (2 in this example) by 60 to give the length of time taken in seconds.

Therefore, our calculation would be:

Speed = Distance/Time

Distance = 60 meters

Time = 60 × 2 seconds = 120 seconds

Therefore,

Speed = 60/120

Speed = 0.5 meters per second

Questions will often give distance in miles and require an answer in meters per second (or vice versa). In this case, you will be told within the question that there are roughly 1.6 kilometres in a mile, and so simply divide the number of kilometres by 1.6 to calculate the number of miles, or multiply the number of miles by 1.6 to calculate the number of kilometres.

Hints and Tips

If a question mentions a specific conversion (i.e. 1 mile = 1.6 kilometres) then you can be sure that you are expected to make use of it! If you have reached an answer without making use of the formula, you might want to double check to make sure that all of your units are correct.

Learning the formulas and being able to quickly identify which is needed will drastically improve the speed at which speed, distance and time questions can be answered.

Worked Examples

1. On her last run around the park, Katie ran 5km in 25 minutes. Calculate the speed at which she travelled:

A. 150 m/minute

B. 200 m/minute

C. 250 m/minute

D. 300 m/minute

E. 350 m/minute

Solution: Straight away, we should notice that we are given Katie's distance in kilometres, but all of the answers are in meters per second. We know that there are 1000 meters in a kilometre, and so Katie ran:

1000×5 meters = 5000 meters

Speed = Distance/Time

Speed = 5000/25

Speed = 200 m/minute

Therefore, the correct answer is B.

2. The fast train from Town A to City B travels at an average speed of 60 km/h. One journey takes 5 hours. Given that 1 mile = 1.6 kilometres, calculate the distance between Town A and City B.

A. 136.0 miles

B. 155.5 miles

C. 174.0 miles

D. 187.5 miles

E. 201.0 miles

Solution: Straight away we should notice that we have been given speed in km/h, but all of the answers are in miles.

1 mile = 1.6 km

Therefore 1 km = 1/1.6 miles

Therefore 60 km/h = 60/1.6 mph

60 km/h = 37.5 mph

Speed = Distance/Time

Distance = Speed × Time

Distance = 37.5 × 5

Distance = 187.5 miles

The correct answer is therefore D.

2. Percentages

Questions revolving around percentages also occur frequently throughout the UCAT. There are a number of different formulas here that should be learnt to cover a wide variety of different percentage-related questions that might be asked.

There are 6 types of percentages questions that you should be aware of:

1. Finding the percentage of a number

Finding the percentage of a number is relatively easy:

1. First, turn the percentage into a decimal.

2. Next, multiply the decimal by the number you are finding the percentage of.

To turn a percentage into a decimal, divide the percentage by 100.

Essentially, percentage means out of a 100.

So, 15% written as a decimal = 15/100 = 0.15

So, if we are trying to find 15% of 100, multiply 100 with 0.15 = 15

Likewise, if we are trying to find 15% of 200, multiply 200 by 0.15 = 30

2. Calculating a new number after a percentage increase or decrease

Sometimes we are required to find a new amount after there is a percentage increase or decrease.

For example, we might be told that a pair of shoes usually costs £40, but that it is on sale at 20% off. to calculate the new price, we must:

1. Turn the percentage into a decimal by dividing it by 100.
2. Multiply the decimal by the number you are finding the percentage of:
3. (A). ADD this new number onto the original price if there was a percentage INCREASE.
3. (B). SUBTRACT this new number from the original price if there was a percentage DECREASE.

So, if we are trying to calculate the new price of the shoes, we first turn the percentage into a decimal: 20% = 20/100 = 0.2

We then multiply this by the original price: 0.2×40 =8

A quick way to work this out would be 2 X 40 = 80, and then dividing by 10 = 8.

Finally, we then subtract this number from the original price (we subtract it because the price has been reduced, so we are dealing with a percentage decrease).

Answer = 40−8 = 32

The new price is therefore £32.

3. Expressing one number as the percentage of another

Sometimes we will be asked to express one number as the percentage of another:

For example, we might have to express x as a percentage of y, or maybe we might have to express 5 as a percentage of 10.

1. First we divide the first number by the second (divide x by y).
2. Next, we multiply this number by 100

Effectively: First Number/Second Number ×100

So, if we are expressing 5 as a percentage of 10, we start by dividing 5 by 10 = 5/10 = 0.5

We then multiply this number by 100: 0.5×100 = 50%

Therefore 5 is 50% of 10.

4. Finding the original number after there has been a percentage increase or decrease

Sometimes we will be told that an unknown number has experienced a percentage change to create a new, known number. We will then have to work out the original number.

For example, imagine that we are told that a dress is on sale at 30% off and that the sale price is £35.

We must work out the original price before the sale:

1. Write down the new cost as a percentage of an original cost.
2. Divide to find out what 1% of the original cost was.
3. Multiply by 100.

Let's work through our example:

First, we must write down the new cost as a percentage of the old cost.

The dress costs 30% less than it originally cost.

Normal cost of the dress = 100%

A 30% decrease equals 70% of the original cost (because 100−30=70).

Therefore £35 is 70% of the original cost. Now set up a ratio to work out 1%.

£35 = 70%

? = 1%

Therefore 1% of the original cost:

1% = 35/70

1% = 0.5

We know that the original cost of the dress is 100%.

£0.5 = 1%

? = 100%

To go from 1% to 100%

100% of the original cost therefore equals:

= 0.5×100

= 50

Therefore, the original cost was £50.

5. Calculating a percentage change

Sometimes we are given the original number and a new number and told to calculate the percentage change.

For example, imagine that we are told that a watch cost £150 last year but rose in price to £210 this year. We must calculate the percentage change:

There is one simple formula to use here:

Percentage Change= [(New Number − Old Number)/Old Number] ×100

If the resulting number is positive, then there has been a percentage increase.

If the resulting number is negative, then there has been a percentage decrease.

Therefore, the percentage change of our watch is: (210-150)/150×100

60/150 = 0.4

0.4 x 100 = 40

Therefore, there has been a 40% increase in the cost of the watch.

6. Calculating compound interest

Compound interest occurs where a number undergoes a series of concurrent percentage changes. After each change, the new number becomes the next 'original number' when calculating the next percentage increase.

Things become a little more complicated here, but we only need to use a single formula to calculate compound interest.

New Amount=Original Amount $\times (1+r/100)^n$

Where:

r = the percentage change

n = the number of concurrent changes

Let's work through an example:

A loan shark lends Harry £100 and charges compound interest at 1% per day. Harry takes 5 days to pay the loan shark back. Calculate how much Harry must pay back.

Here we can see that:

r = 1%

n=5

Plugging these numbers into the formula, we see that:

New amount = $100 * (1 + 100)^5$

New amount = 105.101005

New amount = £105.10

Worked Examples

1. Claire is looking to purchase a new dress that costs £140. The dress shop is having a promotion whereby all stock costs 30% less than advertised. Calculate the new cost of the dress.

A. 88   B. 98   C. 102   D. 111   E. 125

Solution: Here we are calculating a new number after a percentage increase or decrease.

First, we must turn the percentage into a decimal by dividing it by 100.

$30/100 = 0.3$

Next, we multiply the original number by this decimal.

$0.3 \times 140 = 42$

Finally, because this is a percentage decrease, we subtract this value from the original price to find the new price:

$140 - 42 = 98$

The answer is therefore B.

2. Last year Barry's business made $35,000 in profit. This year it made $105,000. Calculate the percentage increase from last year to this year.

A. 50%   B. 100%   C. 150%   D. 200%   E. 250%

Solution: For this question we simply use the percentage change formula:

Percentage Change = (New Number−Old Number)/Old Number×100

Percentage Change = 105000−35000/35000×100

$70000/35000 = 2$

$2 \times 100 = 200$

Percentage change = 200%

The answer is therefore D.

3. Greg deposits £100 into a savings account that offers 1.5% compound interest annually. Calculate, to the nearest pound, how much money he will have in his account after 3 years, assuming there are no withdrawals.

A. 105   B. 110   C. 115   D. 120   E. 125

Solution: Here we must use our formula for calculating compound interest.

New Amount = Original Amount × $(1 + r/100)^n$

Where:

r = the percentage change

n = the number of concurrent changes

New amount = $100 \times (1+1.5/100)^3$

New amount = 104.5678...

New amount = £105 (nearest pound)

The correct answer is therefore A.

4. A sports shop is having a promotion whereby if you purchase two items together, the cheapest item will cost 40% less and the more expensive item will cost 10% less. Esmerelda wishes to purchase a bike for £250 and a set of skis for £200. How much will she have to pay for both items?

A. £305   B. £345   C. £370   D. £405   E. £450

Solution: This question requires two separate percentage change calculations to be made.

We will first calculate the cost of the cheapest item, the skis, which cost £200 reduced by 40%.

Here we are calculating a new number after a percentage increase or decrease.

First, we must turn the percentage into a decimal by dividing it by 100.

40/100=0.4

Next, we multiply the original number by this decimal.

0.4×200=80

Finally, because this is a percentage decrease, we subtract this value from the original price to find the new price:

200−80=120

The skis will therefore cost £120.

Now we turn to the bike which cost £250 reduced by 10%

Again, we are calculating a new number after a percentage increase or decrease.

First, we must turn the percentage into a decimal by dividing it by 100.

10/100=0.1

Next, we multiply the original number by this decimal.

0.1×250=25

Finally, because this is a percentage decrease, we subtract this value from the original price to find the new price:

250−25=225

The bike will therefore cost £225.

In total the items will cost £120 + £225 = £345.

The correct answer is therefore B.

3. Ratio & Proportion

A ratio is the relationship between two values which gives the size of one value relative to the other value.

For example, if there are twice as many apples as there are oranges, the ratio of apples to oranges would be 2:1.Similarly, if we know that there are 5 pears and 2 pineapples, the ratio of pears to pineapples would be 5:2.

Ratios are useful because if we know the value of one item and are given its ratio to a second item whose value is unknown, we can calculate the value of that second item.

For example, if we are told that there are 10 melons and the ratio between melons and grapes is 10:17, we know that there must be 17 grapes.

1. Reducing a ratio to its simplest form

It is often useful to write a ratio in its simplest form; that is, by reducing each number within the ratio to the smallest possible whole number. The best way to do this is to:

Divide each value within the ratio by their highest common factor.

The highest common factor is the highest factor that both of the values share.

For example, let's say that we have the ratio 10:5.

We know that the factors of 10 are 1, 2, 5 and 10.

We know that the factors of 5 are 1 and 5.

The highest common factor is therefore 5.

Dividing both numbers within the ratio by 5 gives a new ratio of 2:1.

Therefore 10:5 is the same as 2:1, except the ratio has been reduced to its simplest form.

Ratios will not always need to be reduced to their simplest form, but there will be occasions where it is beneficial to do so.

2. Using a ratio to calculate an unknown value

Calculating an unknown value using a known value and a ratio is relatively simple:

Unknown Value = Known Value/Known Ratio Number × Unknown Ratio Number

So, for example, imagine that we are told that there are 10 boys in a class and that the ratio of boys to girls is 2:5. We must calculate the number of girls in the class.

Unknown value = number of girls

Known Value = number of boys

Known ratio number = ratio number for boys = 2

Unknown ratio number = ratio number for girls = 5

Question stem says: 10 boys: ? girls

We have been told ratio is 2: 5

So, 10 boys represents 2 parts. 1 part = 5 boys.

If the ratio is 2:5 then 5 parts = 5 x 5 = 25

There are, therefore, 25 girls in the class.

Advanced Techniques

1. Simplifying ratios containing decimals or fractions

Sometimes ratios will be written to include decimals or fractions. For example, 2.5 : 5.5 and 2/5 : 3/10 are both ratios.

These can be tricky to deal with and it is a lot easier to simplify the ratio before performing calculations.

To simplify a ratio involving decimals, keep multiplying both sides by 10 until you are left with whole numbers (Remember that both sides of the ratio must be multiplied by 10 the same number of times!)

Then, reduce the ratio to its simplest form as you normally would.

If our ratio is 2.5 : 5.5 we multiply both sides by 10 to give a new simpler ratio of 25 : 55, which we can then reduce accordingly.

To simplify a ratio involving fractions, give both fractions the same common denominator and then multiply by that common denominator.

Then, reduce the ratio to its simplest form as your normally would.

If our ratio is 2/5 : 3/10, we convert both fractions to have the same common denominator.

We are left with 4/10 : 3/10.

We then multiply both sides by our common denominator to give 4 : 3. If it were possible to reduce this accordingly, we would then do so.

2. Proportional division

Some questions will give a total number and state that it is to be shared to a specific ratio.

For example, we might be told that in total there are 30 children in a class and that the ratio of boys to girls is 2 : 1. Here we must calculate 2 unknown values: the number of girls and the number of boys.

First, we must 'slice' the ratio up into individual chunks. Each number separated by ':' is one slice. So, if the ratio is 3 : 7, there are two slices. One slice is 3, one slice is 7.

If the ratio is 3 : 7 : 7, there are 3 slices. One slice is 3, one slice is 7 and one slice is 8.

Next, we calculate the sum of the slices.

So, if our ratio is 2 : 1, the sum of the slices is 2 +1 which equals 3.

If our ratio is 3 : 7 : 8 the sum of the slices is 3 + 7 + 8 which equals 18.

We then divide the total number given in the question by this sum of the slices.

The total number of children in the class is 30. 30/3 = 10

Next, take the resulting value and multiply it by each 'slice' of the ratio to give a value that corresponds to the number within that slice.

The ratio of boys to girls given to us was 2 : 1.

The total number of boys is therefore 10×2 = 20.

The total number of girls is therefore 10×1 = 10.

Check that the sum of your two answers is equal to the total given in the question.

Hints and Tips

- Reducing a ratio to its simplest form can make it easier to calculate an unknown value in your head; imagine that we are given a ratio of 116:232 (which can be simplified to 1:2). It is a lot easier to mentally multiple something by 2 than it is by 116!

- Questions will often incorporate ratios and proportions as a small part of a larger question; the question might primarily require speed, distance and time calculations, but one part of one question might require ratio work as an added element.

- When using formula, sometimes we do not need to simplify ratios when we are inputting numbers into a calculator. However, it might be the case that simplifying the ratio allows for the answer to be quickly answered using mental maths which can save a great deal of time. See Worked Example 1 for an example of this.

Worked Examples

These questions are designed to help you get to grips with the calculations stated above, and do not necessarily represent the questions you will see in the exam directly; sometimes, examination questions will require use of one of these calculations within the context of a broader problem question.

1. The ratio of strawberries to tomatoes sold at a market stall is 4:12. 96 tomatoes were sold. Calculate how many strawberries were sold.

A. 32　　　　　B. 45　　　　　C. 56　　　　　D. 57　　　　　E. 62

Solution: This question requires us to calculate an unknown value from using a ratio. The formula we must use is as follows:

Unknown Value = Known Value/Known Ratio Number × Unknown Ratio Number

Our known value is the number of tomatoes sold, 96.

Our unknown value is the number of strawberries sold.

Our known ratio number is 12.

Our unknown ratio number is 4.

Unknown Value = 96/12 x 4

Unknown value = 32

Therefore 32 strawberries were sold and so the answer is (a).

Note that because we are plugging numbers into a formula, we do not need to simplify this ratio. However, if we simplify the ratio to 1:3 it becomes a lot easier to calculate the answer using mental maths, which will drastically increase the speed at which the question is answered; there were 3 times as many tomatoes sold than strawberries and so we can easily divide 96 by 3 in our heads to reach the correct answer of 32.

If you find it tricky to wrap your head around the formula. Let's work through it step by step: strawberries to tomatoes sold at a market stall is 4:12. 96 tomatoes were sold

Strawberries : Tomatoes

Ratio given 4:12

? Strawberries : 96

12 parts represents 96

Therefore, 1 part = 8

If strawberries are represented by 4 parts.

4 x 8 = 32

2. Express the ratio 6.6 : 9.9 in its simplest form.

A. 1:3   B. 2:3   C. 3:4   D. 3:2   E. 3:1

Solution: To simplify a ratio that involves decimal points, we must keep multiplying both sides by 10 until we are left with whole numbers.

6.6 : 9.9

Becomes

66 : 99

We then divide each number by the highest common factor.

The highest common factor is 33.

We are left with a ratio of 2 : 3.

3. Fred the fisherman catches 204 fish on a particular fishing trip. He catches a variety of mackerel, Pollock and bass, to the ratio of 2: 3 : 7. Calculate the number of pollock that he caught.

A. 36   B. 44   C. 45   D. 48   E. 51

Solution: This question requires us to make use of proportional division. First, we must slice the ratio into distinct chunks. Here we have three slices: 2, 3 and 7.

Next, we calculate the total of these slices: 2 + 3 + 7 = 12

We now divide the total number of fish caught by this total number of slices: 204/12 = 17

We know that 1 slice represents 17 fish and so we multiple the pollock 'slice' by 17 to give the answer: 3 ×17 = 51

51 pollock were therefore caught, and so (e) is the correct answer.

4. Conversion of units

Often, questions are given in one unit but the answers are in a different one. Therefore, it is very important to pay close attention to units or risk choosing the wrong answer.

An example of a question that requires unit conversion at the end of a calculation is as follows: Tom runs 10 miles in 60 minutes. Given that 1 mile = 1.6km, calculate the speed at which Tom ran in km/h.

In this question, we would first use our speed, distance and time formulas (see Speed, Distance and Time) to calculate that Tom ran at a pace of 10 miles/h.

Once this calculation has been made, we must convert 10 miles/h into km/h to give the correct answer.

Basic Strategy

The topic of conversion of units should be seen as an extension of the topic of ratios and proportions.

When we convert a value from one unit to another, we are essentially expressing the ratio of the two units.

For example, if we are told that 1 mile is equal to roughly 1.6km, the ratio of miles to km is 1:1.6.

Therefore, for every 1 mile, there are 1.6 km and so 10 miles are equal to 16 km.

Given that we are essentially working with ratios, we can simply use the techniques given in Ratio and Proportion to finish the calculation.

It should be noted that a great deal of the time, the ratio given will be 1:x. For example, you might be told that 1 mile is equal to 1.6 km, or that 1 foot is equal to 12 inches. These ratios are very simple to convert but are best explained using an example:

Imagine that we are told that the ratio of miles to km is 1:1.6.

If we need to convert from miles to km, we multiply by 1.6.

If we need to convert from km to miles, we divide by 1.6.

This will work for any ratio expressed as 1:x.

If you know the value that corresponds with '1', multiply by xx to find the corresponding value to xx.

If you know the value that corresponds with 'xx', divide by xx to find the corresponding value to '1'.

Memorising these two simplified formulae will make conversion of ratios of 1:x a great deal faster.

Advanced Techniques

Sometimes units will be made up of multiple components. For example, the unit of speed has two components, distance and time. A speed of 100km/h is an expression that someone can travel 100 km in 1 hour.

In more difficult questions, both units will need to be converted to give the correct answer.

An example of such a question is as follows:

Livy travelled from town A to town B at a speed of 21 km/h. Calculate the speed at which she travelled in m/minute.

In this question we must convert the distance component from kilometres to metres and then the time component from hours to minutes.

We know that 1 km is equal to 1000m. The ratio is therefore 1:1000.

Livy therefore travelled 21 × 1000 metres in 1 hour

= 21,000m in 1 hour

We know that 1 hour is equal to 60 minutes. The ratio is therefore 1:60.

21000/60 = 350

Therefore, Livy travelled at a speed of 350m/minute.

Hints and Tips

A common trap that many students fall into is that they only pay attention to units at the end of a problem; if a question requires more than one calculation to be made, make sure that the units are converted for the first calculation if necessary!

Remember that when converting units of an area of a shape:

1m2 = 10,000cm2(1m2 = 100cm2 × 100cm2 = 10,000cm2)

Worked Examples

1. Derek is looking to book a holiday to America. He has saved £4570 for his trip. Given that $1.00 is worth £0.69, calculate how many dollars Derek will have for his trip.

A. $3277.50   B. $4567.33   C. $6623.19   D. $6985.20   E. $7560.00

Solution: We start by expressing the two currencies as a ratio. 1 dollar = 0.69 sterling

Our ratio of dollars to sterling is therefore 1:0.69

? dollar = £ 4570

To work out dollars we do £4570/0.69

4570/0.69=6623.1884...

Therefore, Derek has $6623.19 available to him and so the correct answer is (C).

2. Luggage on an airplane costs €7 per kg. Tony is an American tourist whose luggage weighs 59.4lbs. Given that €1.00 is equivalent to $1.44, and that 1kg is equivalent to 2.2lbs, calculate how much Tony will have to pay to transport his luggage.

A. £102.65   B. $135.09   C. $250.00   D. $272.16   E. $415.80

Solution: This is a question that requires us to convert two separate units. We will begin with converting the weight of the luggage from lbs to kg: 1 kg = 2.2lbs

Our ratio of kg to lbs is therefore 1:2.2.

Again, because this is a ratio expressed as 1:x1:x we can quickly save time by simply dividing the weight of the luggage in lbs by 2.2. 59.4/2.2=27

The luggage therefore weighs 27kg.

Our first conversion is complete, and so we must now calculate the cost of luggage in Euros.

1 euro = 1.44 dollars

Our ratio of euros to dollars is therefore 1:1.44

Again, because this is a ratio expressed as 1 : x we can quickly save time by multiplying our value for euros by 1.44: 7×1.44 = 10.08

Luggage therefore costs $10.08 per kg.

Now that our two conversions are complete, we can calculate the cost of 27kg of luggage at a rate of 10.08 per kg: 27×10.08 = 272.16

Tony will have to pay $272.16 and so (D) is correct.

5. Probability

Probability is a measure of how likely something is to happen. As probability increases, the event becomes more probable; that is, the event is more likely to occur. The opposite is true as probability decreases; the event is less likely to happen.

Probability can be expressed as either a decimal or a fraction and must be between 0 and 1.
A probability of 1 indicates that something is guaranteed to happen.
A probability of 0 indicates that something will never happen.

1. Calculating probability

There is a simple formula that we use to calculate the probability of something happening:
Probability = Number of ways for something to happen/Total number of results
It is extremely important to note that this formula only works when all of the different options are equally likely to occur. To give an example, when we roll a standard dice, it is equally likely to land on any particular face. This formula could therefore be used to calculate the probability of it landing on any face.
If the dice were misshapen and some faces larger than the others, there would not be an equally likely chance of it falling on each face and so this formula could not be used.

2. Calculating expected frequency

If we are told the probability of something happening, we can calculate how many times we would expect it to happen if we were to perform the action multiple times. For example, if we are told that the probability of a flipped coin landing on heads is 0.5, we can calculate how many times we would expect it to land on heads if we flip it 100 times:
Expected Frequency = Probability × Number of Repetitions
So, in our coin example, the expected frequency of heads would be: 0.5×100 = 50
Expected frequency = 50 times

Advanced Techniques

There are a number of rules that you should be aware of that the probability of multiple events happening. These techniques will work for any number of events, but for simplicities sake we will assume that we are dealing with 2 individual events, 'Event 1' and 'Event 2'.

1. Calculating the probability that ALL events happen - The AND rule

Sometimes we will need to calculate the probability that both 'Event 1' AND 'Event 2' will occur. We must use the following formula:

Probability of Both = Probability of Event A × Probability of Event B

$P(Both) = P(A) \times P(B)$

This formula can be extended to cover more than 2 events; simply continue to multiply by the probability of each further event:

For example, if we are dealing with 4 events, the probability of them, all occurring is:

$P(all) = P(A) \times P(B) \times P(C) \times P(D)$

So, for example, imagine we have a standard 6 sided die, which we roll twice. We can calculate the probability that the die will land on 1 BOTH times using our formula:

$P(Both) = 1/6 \times 1/6$

$P(Both) = 1/36$

It is important to note that this will only work when the events are independent; that is to say, that the result of one event will not affect the probability of the second event.

2. Calculating the probability that AT LEAST ONE event happens - The OR rule

Sometimes we will need to calculate the probability that either 'Event A' OR 'Event B' will occur. This rule can only be used on mutually exclusive events; that is to say, events that cannot occur at the same time.

Probability of Either Event = Probability of Event A + Probability of Event B

$P(Either) = P(A) + P(B)$

So, for example, imagine that we roll a 6 sided dice. There are 6 independent events that might occur (it might land on any of the 6 faces). The probability that it lands on either a 1 or a 2 would be:

$P(Either) = 1/6 + 1/6$

$P(Either) = 2/6 = 1/3$

This formula will work for a large number of mutually exclusive events; simply continue to add the probabilities together.

Worked Examples

1. Tom rolls 3 standard six-sided, unbiased dice. Calculate the probability that the first and third dice land on 6, whilst the second lands on a 1.

A. 1/2   B. 1/18   C. 1/72   D. 1/216   E. 1/300

Solution: Here we must use the AND rule to calculate the probability.

P(all 3) = P(A) × P(B) × P(C)

P(all 3) = 1/6 × 1/6 × 1/6

P(all 3) = 1/216

The correct answer is therefore (D).

2. Annie rolls a single, fair 50 sided dice (each side is equally as likely to occur). Calculate the probability that she rolls a number between 1 and 25 inclusive.

A. 1/3   B. 1/2   C. 2/7   D. 4/7   E. 1/4

Solution: Here we must use the OR rule to calculate the probability.

P(Either) = P(A)+ P(B)

P(Either) = P(1) + P(2)+ ... P(24) + P(25)

The probability of landing on any face is 1/50, therefore the probability of landing on a 1 is 1/50, the probability of landing on a 2 is 1/50 etc. Because all of the probabilities are the same here, we can simply multiply 1/50 by 25 (the total number of qualifying events) to save us time. Therefore, the Probability of either is: P(Either) = 1/50 × 25

P(Either) = 1/2

The correct answer is therefore (B).

3. Tony has a big bag of sweets. 50 are blue, 30 are red and 20 are green. Assuming that the probability that he pulls any particular sweet out is the same, calculate the probability that he pulls out a red sweet.

A. 1/10   B. 2/10   C. 3/10   D. 4/10   E. 5/11

Solution: Here we must use our probability formula:

Probability = Number of ways for something to happen/Total number of possible results

Probability = 30/(50+30+20)

Probability = 30/100

Probability = 3/10

The correct answer is therefore (C).

6. Tables & Diagrams

A large number of questions will begin with a table or diagram containing lots of information. Individual questions will then refer back to this and the information provided must be used to correctly answer the question.

The difficulty in answering these types of question will often lie in successfully extracting the correct information from the table or diagram. Other calculations will often be required, but these will revolve around the extracted information; if the wrong information is taken, an incorrect answer will be found.

The information given in tables and diagrams will often need to be used in conjunction with calculations from other topics; for example, a timetable might give the time it takes for a train to travel between various stations, along with the respective distances. A question would require the correct information to be extracted for two particular stations before a speed, distance and time calculation is made to give the speed at which a certain train travels.

There are no formulas to learn for tables and diagrams specifically; the information here seeks to familiarise you with the type of data that might need to be extracted and what questions might look like in the exam.

'Basic' Tables

Example 1

Station	Time of Arrival (24-hour clock)		
	Train A	Train B	Train C
Green Town	05:00	06:00	07:00
Blue Town	05:30	06:30	N/A
Yellow Town	05:45	06:45	N/A
Red Town	06:10	07:10	07:45
Orange Town	06:30	07:30	08:00

1. How long does it take for Train A to travel to Orange Town from its arrival at Green Town (in minutes)?

A. 60   B. 75   C. 90   D. 105   E. 120

Solution: This is a very simple question which requires nothing more than the extraction of data from the timetable. No substantial maths is required. These questions are important to answer in the exam because they take very little time and are generally very easy so if you find that you are running out of time it is definitely worth it to quickly skim the questions to pick up easy marks.All that we need to do to answer this question is note that Train A arrives at Green Town at 05.00 and arrives at Orange Town at 06.30. We can quickly and easily acknowledge that there is a difference of 1 and a half hours which common sense tells us is equal to 90 minutes. (C) is therefore correct.

2. By what percentage is Train C faster than Train B when travelling between Green Town and Orange Town?

A. 30%   B. 33%   C. 40%   D. 50%   E. 66%

Solution: This question requires extraction of information from the table which is then used to calculate percentage increase. We must first read the table and see that it takes Train C 60 minutes to complete the journey whilst it takes Train B 90 minutes.

We then use our formula from Percentages to calculate percentage change:

Percentage Change = [(New Number−Old Number)/Old Number]×100

Percentage Change = (90−60)/90 × 100

Percentage change = (30)/90 × 100 = 1/3 = 33%

Train C is therefore 33% faster and so the correct answer is (B).

Example 2

	Men	Women	Boys	Girls
Enjoy Coffee	5	7	3	2
Dislike Coffee	3	2	11	4

Kathy surveyed a number of people as to whether they enjoyed or disliked drinking coffee. Her results are displayed in the table above.

1. How many people did Kathy survey?

A. 17   B. 25   C. 37   D. 42   E. 50

Solution: Once again, we see that this is a simple question that requires very little maths. These types of question should be prioritized in the exam as they are easy to answer correctly.

Simply adding the 8 numbers given in the table tells us that Kathy surveyed 37 people in total. The correct answer is therefore (C).

2. Calculate the percentage of girls who enjoy drinking coffee (to 1 decimal place).

A. 33.3%   B. 45%   C. 50%   D. 66%   E. 71%

Solution: We need to extract two pieces of information from the table to answer this question: the number of girls who stated that they enjoy drinking coffee and the total number of girls surveyed.

Girls who enjoy coffee = 2

Total number of girls = 2 + 4 = 6

We must apply the formula from Percentages to calculate the percentage of girls who enjoy coffee. As per the tutorial:

To express one number as the percentage of another we:

1. First we divide the first number by the second (divide x by y).

2. Next, we multiply this number by 100

Percentage = First Number/Second Number × 100

Percentage = 2/6 × 100

Percentage = 33.333%= 33.3% (1d.p.)

The correct answer is therefore (A).

Dense Tables

Dense tables are really just an extension of regular tables, except they will often contain a great deal of densely compacted information. The main reason that they deserve their own category is that it will often take longer to extract the relevant information and so under time pressure they are more problematic. It is important to skim these tables for keywords that indicate the relevant data, as spending too much time meticulously trawling through them can easily lead to a time shortage later on. Other than this, the principles of data extraction we use here are exactly the same as before.

Example 1

Content	Sample A	Sample B	Sample C	Sample D	Sample E	Sample F
Iron	55%	44%	22%	27%	7%	91%
Copper	31%	12%	11%	15%	8%	3%
Phosphorous	10%	11%	?%	8%	25%	?%
Silica	3%	13%	8%	17%	24%	0%
Other Materials	1%	20%	50%	33%	36%	6%

The above table shows the content of 6 different samples that were sent to a lab for testing.

1. Calculate the percentage of phosphorous found in Sample C.

A. 9%   B. 11%   C. 13%   D. 15%   E. 0%

Solution: For this question we must quickly identify that the contents of Sample C are given in the fourth column. We cannot simply look for a missing data value, as there is also a missing value under phosphorous for Sample F. We must then calculate the sum of the percentages within Sample C aside from phosphorous: 11 + 22 + 8 + 50 = 91

We then subtract this number from 100%. This is because everything should add up to 100%.

$100 - 91 = 9$

Therefore, the percentage of phosphorous found in Sample C must be 9%, meaning that (A) is the correct answer.

2. Sample A weighs a total of 14g. Calculate the weight of copper within Sample B.

A. 4.02g   B. 4.34g   C. 4.56g   D. 4.67g   E. 4.89g

Solution: Looking at the table we see that Sample A is 31% copper. We must then use the formula from Percentages to calculate the weight of copper present:

To calculate 31% of 14g:

1. First, turn the percentage into a decimal by dividing by 100.

2. Next, multiply the decimal by the number you are finding the percentage of.

$31/100 = 0.31$

$0.31 \times 14 = 4.3g$

The correct answer is therefore (B).

Multiple Tables or Diagrams

Some questions might involve more than one table or diagram. Sometimes the data given in one will relate to the other and so cross referencing will be required. Whilst adding in additional steps will increase the likelihood of mistakes being made, and will increase the amount of time required to answer the question, the principles at play in these questions will be exactly the same as has been stated previously and so the same techniques should be used.

Diagrams

Sometimes data will be displayed in some form of visual diagram rather than a table. We use the exact same principles here as we would with a table, however; the diagram will contain information that we must extract and then use to perform a specific calculation. As with regular tables, there will be questions that require little to no maths, and once again these easy questions should be prioritised.

These diagrams might come in many different forms; how they look is of little importance. The key idea is to be able to quickly identify the relevant information that they hold.

Example 1

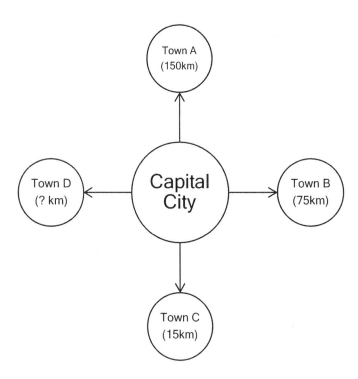

The diagram above displays the distance between a capital city and various surrounding towns.

1. Rav is training for a marathon. He is able to run from the Capital City to Town C and back in 5 hours. Calculate his average speed.

A. 5 km/h   B. 6km/h   C. 7km/h   D. 8km/h   E. 9km/h

Solution: For this question we must make use of the formula given in Speed, Distance and Time. Looking at the diagram we are able to see that Town C is 15km away from the Capital. We know that Rav runs there and back and so the total distance ran is 30km (a common error here might be to forget that Rav is running there and back).

Speed = Distance/Time

Speed = 30/5

Speed = 6km/h

The correct answer is therefore (B).

2. Brian is able to cycle from the Capital City to Town D in 3 hours. His speedometer records that he cycles at an average pace of 17km/h. Calculate the distance between the Capital and Town D.

A. 21km   B. 26 km   C. 30 km   D. 45km   E. 51km

Solution: Again, this question relies on the formula from Tutorial 2 - Speed, Distance and Time. Here we are not actually extracting data from the diagram, but instead we are filling in a blank. This type of question occurs fairly frequently.

Speed = Distance/Time

Draw out the formula triangle and cover the part you want (distance).

Distance = Speed × Time

Distance =17×3

Distance = 51km

The correct answer is therefore (E).

It should be noted that this question could very easily be made more difficult by requiring a conversion from kilometres to miles at the end.

7. Geometry

Some questions within the UCAT will require the use of basic geometric formulas. Once memorised, these formulae are quick and easy to use and so it is certainly beneficial to enter the exam with a sound understanding of what they are and how to use them. The less time that is spent trying to recall a formula in an exam, the more time there will be to answer questions.

Formulae

There isn't a great deal to say when it comes to the level of geometry required for the UCAT; learn the formulae below and practice using them until you are comfortable being able to recall them from memory and rearrange them as needed.

Perimeters

Perimeter of a polygon = sum of all sides

Circumference of a circle = $2 \times \pi \times r$

Areas

Area of a quadrilateral = base × height

Area of a triangle = 1/2 × base × height

Area of a circle = $\pi \times r^2$

Volumes

Volume of a uniform solid = cross sectional area × height

Volume of a sphere = $4/3\pi \times r^3$

Worked Examples

1. Calculate the area of the triangle shown above.

A. 50 cm2   B. 75 cm2   C. 100 cm2   D. 125 cm2   E. 150 cm2

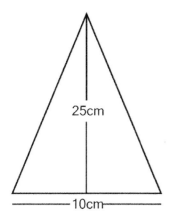

Solution: Here we must recall the formula for the area of a triangle:

Area of a triangle = 1/2 × Base × Height

Area = 12×10×25

Area = 125cm2

The correct answer is therefore (D).

2. Calculate the area of a circle that has a diameter of 44cm.

A. 370п   B. 390п   C. 398п   D. 422п   E. 484п

Solution: Here we must recall the formula to calculate the area of a circle:

Area of a circle = п × r2

Note that we have been given the diameter of the circle; we must half this to find the radius.

Area = п(44/2)2

Area = п × 22 x 2

Area = 484п

The correct answer is therefore (E).

If the answer was looking for a figure. You can use 3.14 as an estimate of Pi.

Practice Questions

As with the VR questions - you can use this as practice or come back to it later for a targeted mock test!

Set 1

A small entertainment store is having its end-of-year annual review of sales of DVD and Blu-ray stock. The graph below shows the number of units of DVD and Blu-ray stock sold each month in 2014.

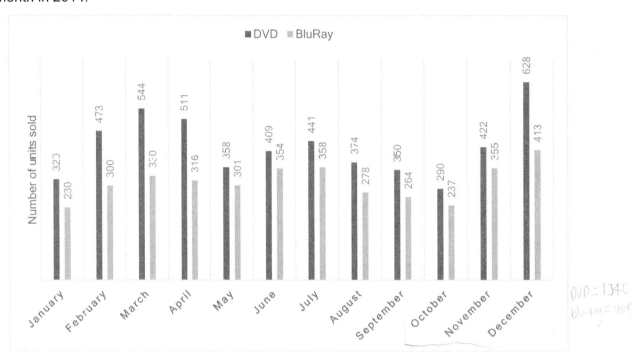

DVD = 1340
blu-ray = 1005

1. Approximately how many DVD and Blu-ray units were sold over the year. Choose the closest figure.

A. 2500   B. 4000   C. 5500   D. 7000   E. 8500

2. In the final quarter of the year, how many more DVD units were sold compared with Blu-ray units?

A. 335   B. 345   C. 355   D. 370   E. 390

3. In December, what is the percentage increase of DVD unit sales compared with Blu-ray unit sales?

A. 44%   B. 52%   C. 66%   D. 68%   E. 70%

4. In January and February, a third product was also sold: USB drives. 77 units were sold over these two months. What fraction, approximately, of total sales of the 3 products were USB drives for January and February?

A. 1/28   B. 3/20   C. 2/36   D. 4/30   E. 2/24

A pharmaceutical company is reviewing the price fluctuations of two of its cancer therapy drugs over the past 5 years.

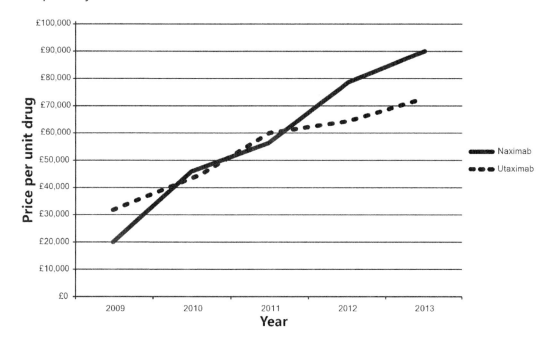

1. How much more did Naximab cost in 2012 than 2010?

A. 26,000   B. 32,000   C. 35,000   D. 38,000   E. 42,000

2. As a percentage, how much more did Utaximab cost in in 2011 than 2009?

A. 75%   B. 80%   C. 87%   D. 100%   E. Unsure

3. Which of the following demonstrated the largest percentage increase from the previous year?

A. Utaximab 2013

B. Utaximab 2012

C. Naximab 2011

D. Naximab 2012

E. Can't say

4. In 2011, a hospital in London ordered both Naximab and Utaximab in the ratio 3:5. In total, they ordered 600 drugs. How much did they pay for Utaximab in millions?

A. 18   B. 19.5   C. 21   D. 22.5   E. 23

Set 3

Jonathan and a few of his friends decided to take a trip up to Scotland from London. The entire journey by car took 6 hours 40 minutes, and this included two stops for petrol, lasting roughly 5 minutes each, and a lunch break lasting 30 minutes. The car's odometer before the journey displayed a value of 1203 miles, and as the group arrived, it displayed 1503 miles.

1. What the average speed the car was travelling at from London to Scotland?

A. 40mph   B. 45mph   C. 50mph   D. 55mph   E. 60mph

2. If there are 1.6 kilometres in a mile, how many kilometres did the group travel in total?

A. 460 km   B. 465 km   C. 470 km   D. 475 km   E. 480 km

3. Another friend ended up taking the train instead, with the total journey taking 2 hours 30 minutes (roughly over the same distance). How much faster was the speed by train than by car, as a percentage increase?

A. 120%   B. 130%   C. 140%   D. 150%   E. 160%

4. In terms of pricing of the journey, the car's petrol costs was shared equally between 4 people. The car used up 32 litres of petrol for the whole journey, and the group paid 120p per litre of petrol. The friend who took the train paid 40 pounds for his ticket. How much more did the friend who took the train end up paying compared to a person who travelled by car?

A. £19.50   B. £25.40   C. £29.30   D. £30.40   E. £31.50

A kickboxing team were required to check the weights of their entrants before a competition.

Student	John	James	Tom	Chris	Josh
Weight	10 stone 9 lb	9 stone 7 lb	84 kg	100 kg	72 kg

1 kg = 2.2 lb

1 stone = 14 lb

1. In lb, how much does James weigh?

A. 120 lb   B. 127 lb   C. 130 lb   D. 133 lb   E. 138 lb

2. In stone and pounds, how much does Tom weigh?

A. 12 stone 12 lb

B. 13 stone 3 lb

C. 13 stone 2 lb

D. 13 stone 5 lb

E. 14 stone 1 lb

3. What is the total weight of all the boys, in kg?

A. 215 kg   B. 265 kg   C. 384 kg   D. 390 kg   E. 420 kg

4. As a percentage, how much heavier is Chris compared to the average of the 5 boys?

A. 20%   B. 30%   C. 40%   D. 50%   E. 60%

Set 5

James and Melissa decided to take separate holidays this summer. James ended up going to Tokyo, and Melissa, who lives in France, took a flight to New York. The flight times table shows the arrival and departure times of their planes at their respective destinations. There is a period of airport transit waiting time between intermediate cities. Note that all flight times indicated in the table are local, and a table of the time differences between cities when London is at 00:00 (midnight) is shown.

James's Flight Timetable

London Departure	Hong Kong Arrival	Hong Kong Departure	Tokyo Arrival
Tuesday 06:00	Wednesday 0:00	Wednesday 03:00	Wednesday 04:00

Melissa's Flight Timetable

Paris Departure	Toronto Arrival	Toronto Departure	New York Arrival
Tuesday 09:00	Tuesday 13:00	Tuesday 15:00	Tuesday 16:00

City time differences

London	Hong Kong	Tokyo	Paris	Toronto
Sunday 00:00	Sunday 08:00	Sunday 09:00	Sunday 01:00	Saturday 19:00

1. How long was Melissa's flight from Paris to Toronto?

A. 4 hours   B. 5 hours   C. 7 hours   D. 9 hours   E. 10 hours

2. What was James' total journey time from London to arriving in Tokyo?

A. 12 hours   B. 13 hours   C. 14 hours   D. 15 hours   E. 16 hours

3. In terms of total flying time, how many more hours did James or Melissa spend on the plane compared to each other?

A. 1 hour   B. 2 hours   C. 3 hours   D. 4 hours   E. 5 hours

4. Both Melissa and James were on Boeing 747s for both legs of their flights to their respective destinations, which uses approximately 4 litres of fuel every second. What is the difference in total fuel usage of the planes for the entire outward journey taken by Melissa and James?

A. 10,200 L   B. 14,400 L   C. 18,400 L   D. 22,800 L   E. 28,800 L

Set 6

Below shows a pie representation of the distribution of the total cohort of incoming medical students for 2015 in Japan according to different medical school types. There are roughly 10,000 medical students in the incoming 2015 cohort. There is also a corresponding pie chart displaying the proportion of first choice pre-term society subscriptions distributed among the new cohort.

Distribution of 2015 student cohort among medical school types

Distribution of first-choice society subscriptions across 2015 student cohort

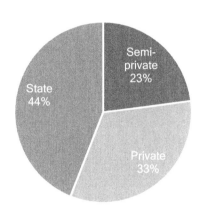

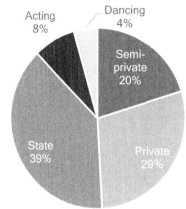

1. How many more students are going to state medical schools than private medical schools?

A. 900   B. 1000   C. 1100   D. 1200   E. 1300

2. If a third of the incoming private medical school cohort are subscribed to sport societies, how many students are subscribed to sport at semi-private and state schools?

A. 1900   B. 2700   C. 2900   D. 3100   E. 3300

3. If the ratio of private to semi-private to state medical school cultural society subscribers was 1 : 4 : 7, how many students subscribed to a cultural society at a state university?

A. 1900   B. 2000   C. 2100   D. 2200   E. 2300

4. Approximately 100 state medical school students that selected music as their first-choice society subscription were unaccounted for in the data above. Given that a quarter of state medical school students were subscribed to a music society, what is the percentage increase in state medical school music society subscribers if we account for the extra number of students?

A. 8%   B. 9%   C. 10%   D. 11%   E. 12%

John is a gardener and has been tasked with laying down grass for his local countryside council. He must fill 0.5 acres of land and has been supplied with grass turf squares, each with a thickness of 7 cm and a side length of 0.64 m.

1 acre = 4046 m2

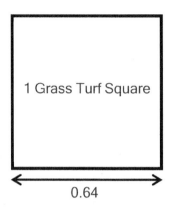

1 Grass Turf Square

0.64

1. What is the area of each grass turf square supplied to John, in m²?

A. 0.29   B. 0.35   C. 0.37   D. 0.39   E. 0.41

2. How many grass turf squares does John need to completely cover the entire piece of land?

A. 4932   B. 4933   C. 4934   D. 4935   E. 4946

3. John decides to redo an area of the land. He takes out 0.58 m³ worth of grass turf squares. How many grass turf squares did he take out?

A. 16   B. 17   C. 18   D. 19   E. 20

4. The council decide to insert a circular fountain to commemorate the town's history. A circle is to be dug for the fountain and has a radius of 6 m. What area of the land will be left after the fountain is inserted, in m²?

(Use Pi to 2 decimal figures: 3.14)

A. 1850   B. 1910   C. 1950   D. 2010   E. 2110

Set 8

Below is a map of four large cities in Switzerland and the distances between them.

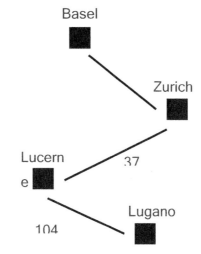

1. It takes 3.5 hours by train from Lugano to Lucerne. At what speed is the train travelling?

A. 29.7 mph   B. 30.5 mph   C. 33.3 mph   D. 39.6 mph   E. 40.5 mph

2. If the train travels at an average speed of 15.6 mph, how long would it take to travel from Lucerne to Zurich

and back?

A. 2 hours 22 minutes

B. 3 hours 12 minutes

C. 3 hours 42 minutes

D. 4 hours 38 minutes

E. 4 hours 45 minutes

3. If a train between Zurich and Basel travels at an average speed of 63 kmph, taking 1.5 hours, how far is Zurich from Basel in miles? Take one mile as being 1.6 kilometres.

A. 35.6   B. 44.0   C. 52.2   D. 59.1   E. 60.5

4. Lugano is at an altitude of 273 meters, whilst Lucerne is at an altitude of 526 meters. The temperature decreases by 0.1°C for every 50 meters gain of altitude. The temperature increases by 1°C for every half hour in the morning. If a train departs Lugano at 08:20, and the temperature on departure is 11.6°C, what will the temperature be on arrival in Lucerne at 11:49?

A. 11.5°C   B. 15.9°C   C. 18.1°C   D. 19.2°C   E. 19.5°C

Below shows a ferry timetable between two ports, East Valbride and Logan Point.

Monday to Saturday

Depart East Valbride	Depart Logan Point
06:30	06:40
06:50	07:00
20 min intervals until -	20 min intervals until -
08:50	08:40
09:15	09:00
30 min intervals until -	09:30
20:45	30 min intervals until -
21:10	21:00
21:30	21:20

Sunday

08:45	08:30
30 min intervals until -	30 min intervals until -
20:45	21:00
21:10	21:20
21:30	-

Crossing times are 95 minutes. The return journey is 120 miles. All ferries are required to wait 1 hour and 15 minutes at either port for unloading, refuelling and reloading.

1. Assume a constant speed. At what speed does the ferry travel?

A. 19 mph   B. 26 mph   C. 38 mph   D. 63 mph   E. 76 mph

2. A ferry leaves East Valbride for the first run on Sunday morning. At what time would it depart Logan point for the return journey?

A. 10:30   B. 11:00   C. 11:30   D. 12:00   E. 12:30

3. The ferry captain wants to sail his ferry to Logan point and leave Logan Point at 0900 to begin his return journey to East Valbride. What time must he leave East Valbride?

A. 06:30   B. 06:50   C. 07:20   D. 08:50   E. None

4. Ben has an interview at 10:20 AM on a Tuesday in East Valbride. He lives in Logan point and wishes to arrive at least 30 minutes early. Which ferry is the latest he should catch?

A. 07:40   B. 07:50   C. 08:00   D. 08:15   E. 08:20

Solutions

1. 8500

This is a simple question; however, it is easy to fall into the trap of summing all values together for an exact answer. Just a quick glance at the answer options reveal there is a significant difference between possible answers, and so a rough approximation is sufficient. If we were to add all numbers together, we would get 8856, and thus 8500 would be the closest figure. Alternatively, we could estimate an average of 300 for Blu-ray sales (shown by the black bars), and an average of roughly 400 for DVDs. Multiply these values by 12 and add them together: (300 x 12) + (400 x 12) = 3600 + 4800 = 8400 - hence 8500 is the closest figure.

2. 335

The final quarter of the year includes October, November and December, and the quickest way is to add all the DVD sales together and then subtract the Blu-ray sales: (290 + 422 + 628) - (237 + 355 + 413) = 1340 - 1005 = 335. Alternatively, we could work out the difference for each month and add the differences, however this is slightly less efficient.

3. 52%

The percentage change formula, which allows us to work out percentage increase or decrease, is: Percentage Change = (Change/Original) x 100; thus, in December: (628 - 413)/413 x 100 = 52%.

4. 2/36

First of all, we need to sum up all values for January and February: 230 + 320 + 473 + 300 = 1323. We then need to include the additional USB drive units: 1323 + 77 = 1400. Left with a fraction of 77/1400, we see that 1400 divided by 77 leaves roughly 18, in other words a fraction of 1/18: double this for a rough fraction of 2/36. Note that much of this can and should be done mentally.

1. 32,000

Again, this is a question that can be done simply by pinpointing. We can see that the value for 2012 is roughly 80,000, and the value for 2010 is slightly under 50,000. The rough estimation we're looking for is bit above 30,000, so 32,000 is the closest approximation.

2. 87%

For Utaximab, we can see that the value for 2011 is 60,000, and the value for 2009 is a bit above 32,000. This can be worked out by realising that this is close to a percentage increase of 100% from 2009 to 2011, but not quite. Consequently, 87% is the closest and thus correct answer. The slower method would be to apply the percentage change formula: (60,000 - 32,000)/32,000 x 100 = 87%.

3. Naximab 2012

This is another question that can be done without any maths. From looking at the graph, we can estimate the percentage increase by the slope of the graph and estimating the difference in price per drug: we see that for Naximab 2012, there is a significant and steep jump between 2011 and 2012. The other options given have smaller jumps between consecutive years, and thus d) must be the answer.

4. £22,500,000

This is a simple proportion question, and it will be easier if you note the answers for intermediate steps onto your whiteboard.

Sum of parts = 3 + 5 = 8

1 part = 600/8 = 75

Amount of Utaximab ordered = 5 x 75 = 375

Amount paid = 375 x 60,000 = £22,500,000

Set 3

1. 50 miles per hour

First of all, we need to work out the distance from London to Scotland: 1503 - 1203 = 300 miles (from the car's odometer). Subsequently, we must find the amount of time the car was on the road and can do so by taking way the two petrol stops and lunch break from the entire journey time: 6 hours 40 minutes - [(2 x 5 minutes) + 30 minutes] = 6 hours.

Thus, to work out the average speed the car was travelling, simply use the speed formula:

Speed = Distance / Time

Speed = 300 / 6 = 50 miles per hour.

Generally, as soon as you see the word 'speed' or 'distance', you should immediately consider looking for applications of the Speed = Distance/Time formula.

2. 480 km

First jot down or mentally note the conversion factor: 1.6 km to 1 mile. We know that the group travelled 300 miles (1503 - 1203), thus the conversion is simply as follows: 1.6 x 300 = 480 km

3. 140% increase

We know that the journey by train took 2 hours 30 minutes and over a distance of 300 miles. The train was therefore travelling at a speed of: D/T = 300/2.5 = 120 miles per hour. Using the previous answer for the speed of the car (50 mph), we can work out the percentage increase in comparison to the speed of the train:

Percentage increase = (new value - original value)/original value x 100

(120 - 50)/50 x 100 = 140% increase.

4. £30.40

So, the car used up 32L of petrol and at 120p per L: this equates to 32 x 120p = 3840p, or £38.40. Be careful here, the costs for petrol were shared equally between 4 friends, and so each person travelling by car only paid 38.40/4 = £9.60 for the journey from London to Scotland.

We know the journey by train costs £40.00, and so the person travelling by train paid 40.00 - 9.60 = £30.40 more than a person travelling by car. The final step should be done mentally to save time.

Set 4

1. 133 lb

We can see that James weighs 9 stone 7 lb, and that the conversion factor is 1 stone = 14 lb. Thus:

9 x 14 = 126 lb

126 + 7 = 133 lb

2. 13 stone 3 lb

Tom weighs 84 kg and the conversion factors are: 1 kg = 2.2 lb, 14 lb = 1 stone. Thus:

84 x 2.2 = 185 lb

185/14 = 13.2 = 13 stone 3 lb (0.2 is approximately 3 out of 14 lb). Remember this final step! It's easy to get caught out and go for option c).

3. 384 kg

We have already worked out James's weight in lb - convert that into kg: 133/2.2 = ~60 kg.

Work out John's weight in lb and then kg:

1 stone = 14 pounds therefore 10 stone 9 lb = (10 x 14) + 9 = 149 lb.

= 149/2.2 = 68 kg.(because 2.2 lbs = 1 kg approximately)

Thus, in total:

60 + 68 + 84 + 100 + 72 = 384 kg

4. 30%

Mean: 384/5 = 77 kg

Chris: 100 kg

Difference = 100 - 77 = 23 kg

Percentage change = 23/77 x 100 = 30%

Set 5

1. 10 hours

This question may be intimidating for those of you who don't like working with time differences, but with practice you'll be fine. The first step is to simply find the difference between the departure time and arrival time: 13:00 - 9:00 = 4 hours. The arrival time in Toronto is local, therefore we need to know the time difference in order to take it into account when calculating the journey time. We can see that at 01:00 in Paris, Toronto is at 19:00 on the previous day: 25:00 - 19:00 = 6 hours. Therefore, Toronto is 6 hours behind. Factor this into our figure above: 4 hours + 6 hours = 10 hours total journey time.

2. 13 hours

This question is quick - make sure you don't waste time working out the times between each city: all you need is the arrival time for the final destination, Tokyo, and the departure time from London. Take into account the time differences at the very end of your calculation.

James arrived at Tokyo at 04:00 (the next day), and left London at 06:00: (24:00 + 4:00) - 06:00 = 22 hours. Then take into account the time difference between Tokyo and London: 09:00 - 00:00 = + 9 hours (ahead), so 22 hours - 9 hours = 13 hours. The total journey time was therefore 13 hours.

3. 2 hours

We already have the total flying time for James from the previous question, 13 hours. For this question, we need the total flying time for Melissa: 16:00 - 09:00 = 7 hours and taking into account time differences between New York and Paris - (24:00 + 01:00) - 18:00 = - 7 hours. New York is 7 hours behind Paris, thus the total flying time for Melissa is 7 hours + 7 hours = 14 hours. Now all that is left to do is subtract the duration of time they were stopped for whilst in their intermediate cities. James stopped for 3 hours whilst Melissa stopped for 2 hours. Their final time spent on a plane will be 10 hours and 12 hours respectively.

4. 28,800 L

For this question, we have an important piece of information: a plane (Boeing 747) uses 4L fuel/second. We must therefore find the total time the planes were actually flying, and this can be derived from subtracting the total journey time for Melissa and James from the transit waiting time in between legs, which happens to be 2 hours for both Melissa and 3 hours for James. Thus: (James) 13 hours - 3 hours = 10 hours, and (Melissa) 14 hours - 2 hours = 12 hours.

We must then do a conversion to maintain the same time unit - converting seconds to hours will probably be easier to work with. To do so, just multiply by 3600. This is because in 1 minute there are 60 seconds. 60 x 60 = 3600. Therefore, 4L x 3600 = 14,400L fuel used per hour. Because we're finding the difference, we know that there is a (12 hours - 10 hours) 2-hour difference between flying time, and so 2 hours x 14,400 L = 28,800 L fuel usage difference.

Set 6

1. 1100

This is a simple percentage and subtraction question: first calculate the number of students going to state medical schools: 10,000 x 0.44 = 4400; and then the number of students going to private medical schools: 10,000 x 0.33 = 3300. To get the answer, simply subtract: 4400 - 3300 = 1100. An even quicker way would be to mentally subtract 33% from 44% to get 11% and multiply this by 10,000.

2. 1900

First of all, we know there are 3300 private medical students in the incoming 2015 cohort (0.33 x 10,000). A third of this would be 1/3 x 3300 = 1100, and this is the number of private medical students interested in sport. To find out how many students are interested in sport in the other two schools, we need to first find the total number of students subscribed to sport societies in 2015: 0.3 x 10,000 = 3000.You can get this bit of information from the pie chart. Subsequently, 3000 - 1100 = 1900 students are subscribed to sport societies in state and semi-private medical schools.

3. 2100

We know that 3600 students have subscribed to a cultural society (0.36 x 10,000 = 3600). To work out the number of students of students subscribed to a cultural society according to the ratio 1 : 4 : 7, we first add up the ratios, or in other words find the sum of the parts: 1 + 4 + 7 = 12. Subsequently, to find the number of students for each part: 3600/12 = 300. Thus, the number of students subscribed to a cultural society at a state university is 7 x 300 = 2100. Remember to always work out 1 part first in their ratio and proportion questions.

4. 9%

You should be able to do this question in your head: first, we know that 1/4 x 4400 = 1100 state school medical students are subscribed to a music society. We also know that there are an extra 100 state school medical students: 1100 + 100 = 1200. In order to calculate the percentage increase, (change/original) x 100: [(1200 - 1100)/1100] x 100 = 9%

Set 7

1. 0.41 m^2

To work out the area of a square, simply multiply the length by itself:

Area = 0.64 x 0.64 = 0.41 m^2

2. 4,935

We know that the area of 1 square = 0.41 m^2, and that 0.5 acres = 2023 m^2. Thus, 2023/0.41 = 4934.1 (We will need 4945 squares to completely fill the land)

3. 20 squares

Volume of 1 square = 0.07 (remember to convert the units from cm to meters) x 0.41 = 0.029 m^3. Thus: 0.58/0.0287 = 20.2.

4. 1910 m^2

The formula for the area of a circle = Pi x r^2. Thus, 3.14 x 6 x 6 = 113 m^2. We know that the total area of land = 2023 m^2, and so the land left: 2023 - 113 = 1910 m^2

Set 8

1. 29.7 mph

This is another simple question requiring application of the Speed = Distance/Time formula: 104/3.5 = 29.7mph.

2. 4 hours 45 minutes

Rearrange the formula - Time = Distance/Speed. 37/15.6 = 2.37; double this to get the return journey, leaving 4.74. 0.74 is roughly equivalent to 3/4, and 3/4 of 60 minutes is 45 minutes: thus, the answer is 4 hours 45 minutes.

3. 59.1 miles

Here we are given a speed in kmph, but all the answer choices are in miles. First of all, convert the 63kmph into mph by dividing by 1.6 to get 39.4 mph as 1.6 km = 1 mile Then to get the answer simply use our familiar formula distance = speed x time. The distance = 39.4 x 1.5 = 59.1 miles.

4. 18.1°C

The altitude difference is 526 - 273 = 253 metres; this gives a temperature decrease of approximately 0.5°C. The journey takes approximately 3.5 hours, meaning a temperature rise of 7°C. Thus, (11.6 - 0.5) + 7 = 18.1°C.

Set 9

1. 38 miles/hour

We must first convert minutes to hours: 95 minutes = 95/60 = 1.58333 hours. We also know that a single crossing is 120/2 = 60 miles. Thus: Application of the Speed = Distance / Time formula = 60 miles / 1.58333 = 38 miles per hour

2. 12:00

The ferry departs at 08:45 and arrives in Logan point at 10:20 (95 minutes crossing time). It makes the required wait until 11:35 (1 hour and 15 minutes) and is therefore ready for the next return crossing which is at 12:00 (having just missed the 11:30).

3. None of the above

If he wishes to return at 09:00, following a 1 hour and 15 minute wait, the latest he must arrive in Logan point is 07:45. He must therefore leave 95 minutes before this, at 06:10. The answer is thus 'None of the above'

4. 08:00

He must arrive by 09:50. 95 minutes before 09:50 is 08:15. The last ferry before 08:15 is at 08:00.

Abstract

Reasoning

What is 'Abstract Reasoning'?

Put simply, this section tests your ability to identify patterns and sequences. To do this effectively, you will need to be able to distinguish important information from distractors, trial and discard incorrect patterns - all under time pressure.

Why do we have to do AR?

It wouldn't be unfair to say that there are quite a few similarities between this section and a conventional IQ test, but then again, the UCAT exam is a psychometric test - natural ability will always have a role to some extent. However, a good system and good habits will maximise your potential. Other than that, the actual accuracy of this section (or the UCAT) in predicting your future success as a doctor is unknown and probably open to debate, but we won't bore you with the finer details. It's in the exam, so you're going to have to get good at it.

Numbers for this section

- **Time**
  13 minutes total = 1 minute for instructions + 12 minutes for questions
- **Questions**
  50 questions total
  10 sets (5 questions each)
- **4 Question Types**
  - **Type 1 -** Presented with two sets of shapes labelled 'Set A' and 'Set B'. You'll be given a test shape and asked to decide whether the test shape belongs to Set A, Set B, or None.
  - **Type 2 -** You'll be presented with a series of shapes. You'll be asked to select the next shape in the series.
  - **Type 3 -** Presented with a statement, involving a group of shapes. You will be asked to determine which shape completes the statement.
  - **Type 4 -** You'll be presented with two sets of shapes labelled 'Set A' and 'Set B'. You'll be asked to select which of the four response options belongs to Set A or Set B.

Following the 1 minute for instructions, you have 12 minutes to get through 10 sets of shapes. Each set consists of 5 test boxes (questions). You, therefore, have around 1 minute 12 seconds to do each set of 5 questions. The good news is that there can be quite a few easier sets that don't take long at all, so you'll probably have more time for the harder questions. We'll go through the exact timings you should aim to stick to later on in the strategy section.

In this section, you may come across a small number of very difficult questions that you won't be able to do, even if you have all the time in the world - but these are rare. A few extra seconds can make a huge difference for sets that require you to run systematically through a large number of options before you reach a pattern. Thus, a good strategy will ensure you maximise the amount of time spent on harder questions and minimize time wasted on easier questions.

Question Types

For this section, there are four question types and named rather unimaginatively Type 1, Type 2, Type 3 and Type 4 sets.

Things to look out for:
Shape · position
· size · Number
· shade

Type 1 Sets

Here's an example of a Type 1 set:

Set A   Set A

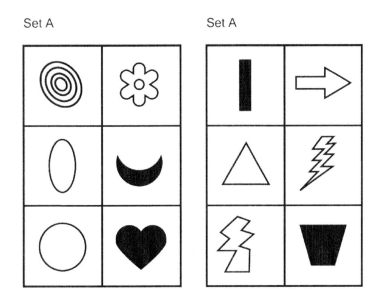

Type 1 sets present you with two collections of shapes named Set A and Set B, and you have to identify a pattern between all boxes within each collection. A 'pattern' is essentially a characteristic (or several characteristics) common to all boxes within a collection. Once you've identified the pattern, you need to apply it to the test box and see if it belongs to Set A, Set B or Neither.

If we take a look at the above example, a common characteristic of all objects in each box of Set A is that they have curved sides. This characteristic holds true for every box in Set A, and so this is a 'pattern'.

The pattern for Set B is usually complementary or opposite to the pattern in Set A: in this particular case, each object in Set B has straight sides.

Once you have the pattern for both Set A and Set B, you then have to apply it to the five test box questions:

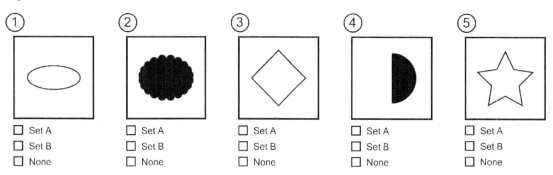

For (1), the object has only curved sides - therefore, it belongs to 'Set A'. Similarly, (2) belongs to Set A. (3) has straight sides, so it belongs to 'Set B'. Interestingly, (4) has both straight and curved sides: this is important - if a test box could belong to both Set A and Set B, the answer is 'None'. Finally, (5) belongs to Set B.

Later on, we'll go into more detail on how we can categorize all these patterns, iron out aspects students commonly find confusing, and work through the best approach for this type of question.

Type 2 Sets

Now, moving on to Type 2 Sets, here's an example:

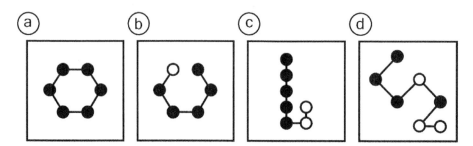

Type 2 sets deal with sequences, which are basically common characteristics that change in a set way as you move along a series of boxes. You're given a series of 4 boxes and must identify the changing characteristics and sequence between the 4 boxes.

In the example above, as we move from one box in the series to the next, a line connected to a shaded circle is added. If you like, this pattern can be further broken down into two characteristics, with the first being the addition of a line and the second the addition of an accompanying shaded circle.

Once you've found the sequence, you're then asked to pick the box that best follows on from this series:

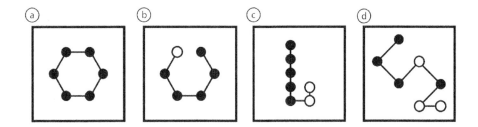

We're expecting a box with five lines and five black circles, along with six circles in total: the answer is therefore (b).

Type 3 Sets

Type 3 sets work by applying rules - here's an example:

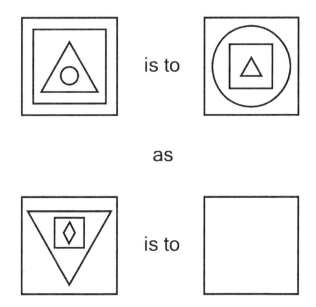

In type 3 sets, you have two statements. The first allows you to identify the changing characteristic i.e. the rule. You must then find the test box that fills the gap in the second statement by applying this rule most closely:

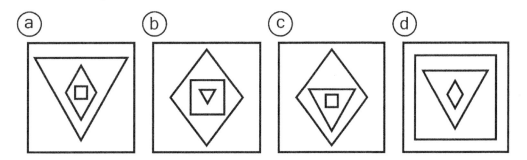

For the example Type 3 set above, a 'position' rule is apparent just by glancing at the first statement. If we follow the small circle in the first box of the statement, we find it becomes the biggest enclosing shape in the second box, whereas the square and triangle shrink to become middle-sized and the smallest of the box respectively. This is the rule, and we can then apply it to our second statement to find the missing box. We're expecting to find the smallest shape in the first box to become the largest enclosing shape, and for the upside down triangle and square to shrink. Indeed, test box (c) matches this perfectly and is, therefore, the correct answer.

Type 4 Sets

Finally, we have Type 4 Sets - here's an example:

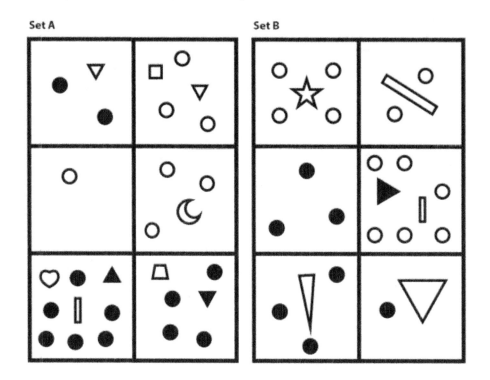

Type 4 sets are basically the same as Type 1 sets: we're given two collections of shapes that each share a common pattern, named Set A and Set B. The only difference is that instead of choosing whether a test box belongs to Set A, B, or Neither as in Type 1 sets, you have to select which of the test boxes fit best with either Set A or Set B.

You would go about finding the pattern for Type 4 sets that same way you would for Type 1 sets. In this example, some of the boxes are much more complicated than others. It is useful to remember that even the simplest box conforms to the pattern we are looking for. The simplest box in Set A contains a single white circle - a characteristic of this circle must contain the pattern we are looking for. Indeed, there's a circle in every box in both Set A and Set B, but the number varies - this may be important. Moreover, some of the circles are white and others are black, this may also be relevant.

Bringing this all together, there is a different total number of circles in each box so this does not help us find the pattern. However, if we incorporate 'shade' into the equation, we find that in Set A, if there's an odd number of circles in a box, the circles are white whereas if there is an even number of circles in a box, the circles are black. The rule for Set B is complementary- if there's an even number of circles in a box, the circles are white whereas if there's an odd number of circles in a box, the circles are black. All other shapes are distractors.

Distribution of question types

Type 1 sets comprise the majority of questions, usually 10 out of 11 sets (50 questions). You'll probably only come across one group of Type 2 or Type 3 sets, or one set of Type 4 questions. When you do, you'll get five different Type 2 or Type 3 sets in a row - or for Type 4 sets, you'll be asked five questions in a row, 'which of the following belongs to Set A/Set B?'.

Preparation Tips

1. Focus on the process rather than the result

When it comes to abstract reasoning questions, it's tempting to move quickly on to the next question when you find the answer. Knowing just the answer won't really help you improve. This goes for everything in the UKCAT, but especially this section. In order see results, you should apply the same systematic process that we teach you in the strategy section over and over again to every question - and whether you get to the answer or not, this approach will in the long-run yield greater results. So make sure that instead of checking the answer and moving on, review how much you stuck to a systematic strategy and whether you applied it properly. The more you do so, and the more you stick to the same approach, the faster you'll get and the more time you'll have left to spend on the harder questions. You'll also pick up the easier to medium patterns much quicker within a few days to weeks. Focus on the process, not the result. Whatever you do, don't stare at the boxes and hope for a pattern to pop into your head.

2. You can be more relaxed with time to begin with

Every section in the UCAT is time pressured, and AR is no different. When you start learning our systematic approach, you'll almost certainly take longer than you will have in the exam. Don't worry, this is normal and just keep at it, focusing on the process we teach you in the strategy section. Over time, you will get faster and start to see a difference. Of course, when doing mock exams, don't be overly relaxed and think you can spend as long as you want, but just bear in mind that it's natural to be slower when internalizing a new strategy in the first few days of practice. Time management is very important, and something you should start doing as soon as you're comfortable with the strategy.

3. Keep track of all the patterns you come across

We'll talk more about this later, but do start keeping a table of all the common to uncommon patterns you come across when practising. This will help you remember and revise the pattern types you come across as you practice. It may be useful to structure your table according to the different pattern categories (which we'll talk about later) and divide it up into easy, medium and hard.

Strategy

Timings

In the abstract reasoning section, it's important not to be held up by difficult questions. Lots of students fall into the trap of wasting time because they think that with a few more seconds they will find the pattern. It is frustrating to have to give up - but if you haven't got it in 30-40 seconds, you probably won't with an extra 10-20 seconds.

Here's a reminder of how much time you're given for AR:

General Timings

Whole section in total.	14 minutes
Questions.	13 minutes
Instructions.	1 minute

Here are the recommended timings for this section:

Recommended Timings

Each set	Under 1 minute
Finding the pattern	Under 30 - 35 seconds
Each test-shape	~ 5 seconds each
Question Type 2, 3 or 4	~ 20 seconds per set

If you work it out, you technically have a bit more than a minute for each set, but we want you to keep it around a minute if you can. This acts as a safety net because you'll probably spend longer than you should anyway and we want to make sure that you have time to get through all the questions. Remember - there may be easy questions at the end and you don't want to miss out on these.

For Type 2 and Type 3 sets, as well as Type 4 sets, you're more pushed for time, although these questions are generally easier to figure out. For Type 1 sets you get one minute for a set of five questions, and you also have a minute for a group of five Type 2 or Type 3 sets (because they are individual questions):

One 'Type 1' Set	1 minute
Five 'Type 2' or 'Type 3' Set	1 minute
One 'Type 2' or 'Type 3' Set	12 seconds

You therefore have around 12 seconds to find the sequence or rule and select the correct answer. If you manage to save some time on the Type 1 questions, you may be able to spend a bit longer, say 15 seconds.

Pattern Categories

For this section, we'll focus on how to best approach the much more common Type 1 sets, later we'll show that you can use the exact same approach for all abstract reasoning question types.

The aim is for you to decide the common pattern in Set A and Set B, and the pattern is a characteristic feature that applies to every single box in the individual set. Once you have a pattern for both Set A and B, you then need to work out which set the test shapes best fits according to the pattern you've just discovered.

Although there are lots of patterns out there, they all fall under a few helpful categories, and we can use these categories to form the basis of our approach.

1. The first category is: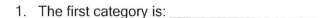

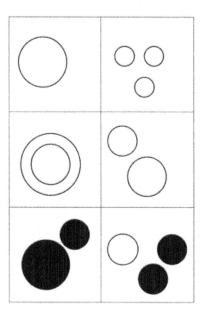

As you can see in the example above, each box contains only circles. This, very simply, is the pattern. A 'shape' pattern is one that has a characteristic that's based on and to do with the object itself; for example, each object in each box may have straight sides, or perhaps all the shapes in a set may be symmetrical.

Just to give you an idea of some of the more common patterns, we've included some tables for the things you should definitely watch out for. Here's a basic list of **shape** patterns you should come across in your practice:

Category	Basic Pattern
Shape	Common shape/object (square, triangle, etc.)
	Common sides:
	- Straight
	- Convex/Concave
	- Regular/Irregular
	Common angles
	Other
	- Symmetrical/Asymmetrical

2. The second category is: _____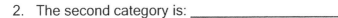

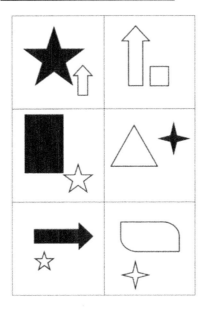

In this example, it should be immediately obvious that there's a big shape accompanied by a small shape in each box, and this is the pattern. Size patterns are generally easy to rule out and pick up - if all the shapes in a box are of equal size, then you can be certain there won't be a size pattern lying around for you to find.

Here are **size** patterns you should be aware of:

Category	Basic Pattern
Size	Common size
	- Big/small (always big shape, etc.)
	Relative size
	- A particular object always larger than another object.

3. The third category is: _____

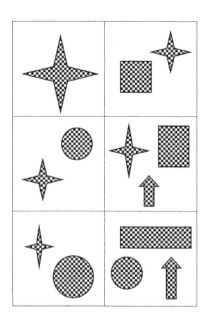

In the example above, all objects in the set have the same shade - this is the pattern. Like size patterns, it should be obvious fairly quickly if there isn't a shade pattern (all shapes will have the same shading).

Here are some **shade** patterns you should know:

Category	Basic Pattern
	Common shade (black/white/shaded pattern)
Shade	- All objects one shade
	- Only certain object shaded

4. The fourth category is: _____

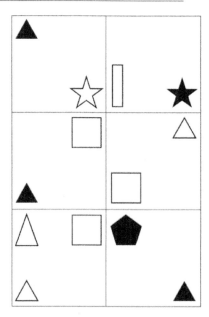

In this set, you can see that the objects within each box are positioned in one of the four corners. Their position in the box is the characteristic here which forms the pattern. In some position patterns, such as this example, the important feature is where the objects are positioned within the box itself (e.g. in the corners, on the left hand side, etc.). However, in some of the more complex position patterns, the key is the positioning of objects relative to each other (e.g. the square is always above the circle). Look out for these tricky position patterns when you practice! Importantly, arrows are a UCAT favourite, and the directions they point towards (up, down, etc.) are often incorporated into position patterns.

Here's a bunch of basic **position** patterns you should be aware of:

Category	Basic Pattern
Position	Object in set position in box - Top/Bottom/LHS/RHS/Corners Object in set position in box - Between shapes - Set rotation Direction of arrows

5. The final and fifth category is _____

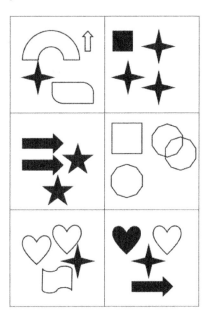

In this example, the pattern is that there are four shapes in each box. Number patterns are common, but not as common as many people think. Lots of students waste time counting for number patterns. This isn't a good habit to get into, especially if there are other more obvious patterns to rule out first.

Here are the most common **number** patterns you could come across:

Category	Basic Pattern
Number	Repeated or characteristic number of:
	- Total shapes
Number characteristics:	- Certain shapes
- Odd	- Sides
- Even	- Enclosed areas/intersections
- Multiples of 3	- Angles

With each number pattern, there could either be a set number of a certain characteristic in each box (3 squares in each box), or one that follows a set number rule, such as there always being an odd number of shapes. Of course, there are some harder number patterns out there, and we'll have a look at those later - but don't get sidetracked with the more difficult questions because they're much rarer and will only leech your valuable time if you get hung up on them.

Now you're familiar with the basic pattern categories, we're going to incorporate these into a strategic approach!.

Approach

The best approach for abstract reasoning is the one that gives you the best chance of finding a pattern in the least time possible. You won't always find the pattern, and that's fine - there are certainly a few difficult questions out there, but as long as you always stick with the same approach and are disciplined enough to flag, guess and skip, you'll be able to maximise your marks on the questions you're more likely to get right.

What you shouldn't do:

1. Stare at the shapes and hope to spot a pattern.

Quite a few test-takers find themselves doing this in AR. Although you may spot an obvious pattern for a simpler question, you're still wasting valuable time, and will most likely miss a more complex pattern.

2. Panic when you can't locate a pattern.

Every set will contain a pattern that will fall into one of the five groups, ensure you're using a strategy that covers the common pattern quickly and efficiently. If you can't seem to locate any patterns, you're probably dealing with a complex dependent pattern. Flag, guess, and move on (there are easier questions up ahead).

3. Start counting for number patterns straight away.

As you practice, you'll soon realise number patterns are common, but it's important to know that the basic patterns are even more common. At the beginning of a set, unless it's obvious there's a number pattern (every box contains 4 shapes, etc.), counting will waste valuable time - ensure you check for simpler patterns first.

4. Spend too long on a set.

Like all subtests, spending a disproportionate amount of time on a harder set means you're sacrificing the time you could use for the easier sets. In AR, by following a systematic approach, you'll be able to identify the majority of patterns not being able to locate a pattern strongly suggests a harder, more complex set, so consider guessing and flagging these on test-day.

Our approach to every set is to systematically run through important characteristics from all five pattern categories, and in the following order:

The mnemonic we use for this is SSSPN.

1. Shape
2. Size
3. Shade
4. Position
5. Number

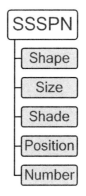

The general step-by-step approach is as follows:

1. **Glance** for any obvious patterns
2. **Compare** the two simplest and most similar boxes using SSSPN
3. **Confirm** in other boxes
4. **Apply** the pattern to the test shapes

Here's the approach in more detail:

Step 1: Glance for any obvious patterns

There are a few patterns that might jump out at you, and with enough practice, you'll be able to pick up more of these patterns. Dedicate five seconds or so at the beginning to just glance at the set – you may spot something, but if you don't, swiftly move on to the next step.

Some of the more obvious patterns you could pick up at first glance include the following:

a) Arrows (if you see an arrow pattern, you should immediately think position pattern)

b) Intersections/Enclosed spaces (these are common and usually indicate a number pattern)

c) Clock faces (the arrows on the clock could be involved in some kind of position pattern)

d) Symmetrical/Asymmetrical shapes (this may not be as obvious until you've seen a few of examples)

Step 2: Compare the two simplest and most similar boxes using SSSPN

For the second step, it's important you pick the two simplest and most similar boxes - this helps stop you from getting caught up with distractors. A shared characteristic you find between two similar and simple boxes in a given set will hold true for every box if it's the correct pattern.

When comparing two boxes within a set, you're looking for and discarding common patterns by running through SSSPN (Shape, Size, Shade, Position, Number), and in that order. The reason we want you to stick with the SSSPN order is simple: patterns under the first three S's (shape, size, and shade) are usually the most visual and more obvious to spot. These patterns can be quickly discarded, so it's more time efficient to start with these categories. Number patterns generally take the longest to tease out, and so it's better to leave this to the end when you've discarded the more obvious patterns.

In situations where you just can't find any patterns when comparing boxes within a set, it might be helpful to compare the simplest box from Set A with the simplest box from Set B. The complementary nature between the two sets means you could spot a difference that might help you find the pattern.

Step 3: Confirm pattern in other boxes

If you find a shared characteristic between two boxes within a set, it goes without saying that you need to check it holds true for other boxes. A pattern must apply to every box in a set. If even one box in the set doesn't follow the pattern you have found, it is incorrect. Having said that, for the sake of saving time, it's usually sufficient to confirm a pattern in three or four boxes (unless you're really unlucky).

Step 4: Apply the pattern to the test shapes

You have your pattern - now you should apply it to the test shapes given (for Type 1 sets), selecting whether it belongs to Set A, Set B or None. If you couldn't find any patterns, just select the same option for all five test shapes, for example 'Set A' (this way, you're bound to get at least some marks). Some of the harder sets will contain multiple patterns, and if pushed for time, just apply whatever you've found - you'll likely get a few marks, and probably won't know if you've missed anything anyway.

Apply SSSPN to your practice

Within the approach given, it's important that you always apply 'SSSPN' to your practice. The more questions you do, the faster you'll be able to bring out and discard patterns under these categories. With any approach we give you, you'll always be slower at the start, but it'll become second-nature as long as you work at it.

Don't worry too much about the more complex patterns because very few people will ever identify them in practice, and it's more worthwhile to get good at spotting the most common patterns first.

Note down the patterns you come across

There's quite a wide range of patterns that can be tested, but all of them can be slotted into one of the five categories. Make sure you keep track of any new patterns you come across during your practice: group them into one of the five categories and try to keep a table you can refer to. You'll increase your chances of locating harder patterns if you note them down and group them properly.

Use the whiteboard to help you

By test-day, you should be confident in using the approach and know it back to front. Even so, many test-takers find it helpful to write down the five categories (SSSPN) onto their whiteboards during the instruction time. The logic is that you'll have something on the whiteboard to get you moving if you panic or get stuck, and you could also use it to note down discarded categories, helping you focus on more likely groups of patterns.

Type 1

Walkthrough

We're going to talk you through the four-step approach by doing a basic, yet helpful, question.

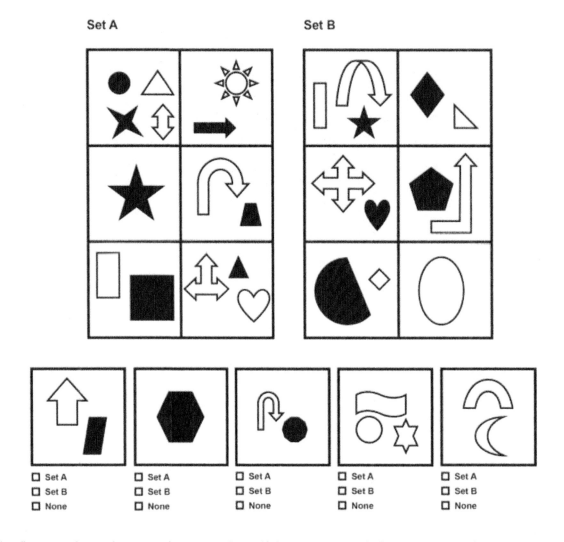

The first step is to glance at the set and see if there are any obvious patterns - but many people will not get this one immediately. Don't waste time staring at the shapes if you haven't arrived at the correct pattern in the first five seconds or so. Move on quickly to selecting the simplest two boxes to compare: we can see straight away that the middle left box is the simplest in Set A, containing only a black star, and we can start by comparing it to the bottom left box.

We should use SSSPN as a framework when comparing boxes: there are no basic shape characteristics common to both boxes; it's also unlikely that there's a size pattern, given that there's only one shape in the middle left box and similarly sized shapes in general. In terms of shade, both boxes contain a black shape, and this could be an important shared characteristic: checking this in other boxes in Set A confirms that every box contains a black shape. Comparison with the simplest box in Set B, specifically the bottom right box as it only contains a single white oval, also reveals that one of the key differences is in the shading. Indeed, all the boxes in Set B contain a white shape, and all boxes in Set A contain a black shape.

We've found our pattern, or at least one of them if the set is more complicated. A position pattern is unlikely given the relatively random placement of shapes in the box, and in terms of number, we can be confident in ruling out the more basic patterns, such as the number of shapes in each box or number of sides. Don't waste time considering more complicated patterns unless you have time to spare.

Our next step is to apply our pattern to the test shapes. The first test shape is tricky and can certainly catch people out - it contains both a black and white shape, and could therefore belong to both Set A and Set B; importantly, if a test shape fits in both Set and Set B the answer is always 'none'. The second test shape contains only a black object, therefore the answer is Set A. Again, the answer to third test shape is 'none' because it contains both a black and white shape. The answer to the fourth and fifth test shapes is Set B because they both contain only white shapes.

Test Shape 1: None
Test Shape 2: Set A
Test Shape 3: None
Test Shape 4: Set B
Test Shape 5: Set B

This example question illustrates how important it is to go for the simplest boxes when comparing and also shows how systematically running through SSSPN can help stop you from missing anything.

Types 2 & 3: Sequences

Basics

Alongside the more common Type 1 sets, for which you're asked to find a pattern for Set A and Set B, you're also given Type 2 and Type 3 sets that require you to look for sequences or rules across a series of boxes (a straight line rotated 90 degrees with every box, etc.).

Type 1 sets consist of five test shape questions per set, however you only get one question for each Type 2 and Type 3 set. Usually, you're given five separate sets of the same type one after the other.

For these sequence sets, you're more likely to come across:
1. Shading Sequences
2. Size Sequences
3. Position Sequences
4. Number Sequences

SSSPN covers any pattern or sequence the UCAT can throw at you, but for sequence sets, you probably won't be given a changing 'shape' category because they are usually patterns that stay the same across all boxes.

Approach

When compared to the Type 1 approach, there are some differences in how you should approach a Type 2 or Type 3 set.

Firstly, you're not really looking for a pattern in these sets because they are sequential, which means there's a changing characteristic. Put simply, you shouldn't be looking for things that stay the same between boxes, but rather characteristics of shapes and objects that change.

The stepwise approach is as follows:
1. **Pick** one aspect and **Follow**
2. **Discard** inconsistent options
3. **Repeat** until answer remaining

Here's the approach in more detail:

Step 1: Pick one aspect and Follow
There's usually more than one sequence, and it's much more effective and time-efficient to discard wrong options as you go along. Firstly, pick one aspect of the first box to follow, which

could be the shade, size, position or number characteristic of a particular object. Usually, this just involves picking an object to follow and noting which of SSSPN changes between boxes.

Step 2: Discard inconsistent options

Once you've discovered a sequence (a diamond rotating 90 degrees with each box, etc.), you should discard any options in the answers that are inconsistent with the sequence. Don't waste time by looking for all the sequences first - a lot of the time, you can get to the answer through discarding without having to find all the sequences between boxes. This is especially relevant for questions where there's a lot going on. You get less time for Type 2 and Type 3 sets, which makes it even more important to discard.

Step 3: Repeat until answer remaining

Continue identifying sequences by picking aspects of the box to follow, and then discarding incorrect options. Do so until you're only left with the answer: the whole process shouldn't take too long, and certainly aim to keep it under 15 seconds.

Walkthrough

Type 2

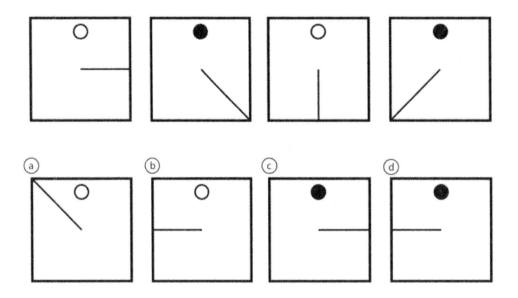

This is a relatively simple illustration of a Type 2 question: these questions can be very simple, which is appropriate because of the little time you get.

1. The first step is to pick one aspect of the box to follow: the circle at the top, for example. As we follow the circle, we can tell there are no changes of 'size', 'position' or 'number': instead, we find it alternates its 'shading' from white to black, and so on - the fifth box in the sequence should therefore have a white circle.

2. We should discard all options that don't have a white circle, which means we can eliminate (c) and (d). We then repeat the process, picking another aspect of the box to follow - this time the line. Clearly, there's a 'position' sequence here: following the line, it rotates 45 degrees clockwise with every consecutive box and touches the corners or middle of each side. We should therefore expect the fifth box to have a horizontal line touching the middle left side: indeed, we can discard (a), and left with (b) as the correct answer.

In the exam, you'll get five of these sets in a row, and these are equivalent to you doing a Type 1 set in a minute.

Type 3

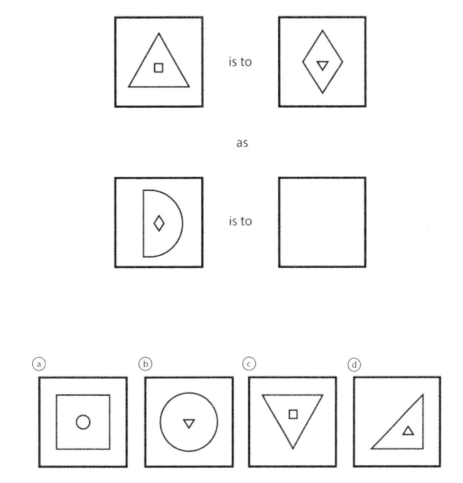

The approach for type 3 sets is the same as that for type 2 sets, although we're given less to work with.

1. Firstly, we pick an aspect of the box to follow, in this case the outer and larger triangle in the first box. The outer shape becomes a diamond in the second box, and there are no changes in 'size', 'shade' or 'position. We're left with a possible 'number' sequence, and indeed, there is a gain of one side as the triangle changes to a diamond. The first box of the next statement contains an outer shape with two sides, and following the sequence from above, the second box should therefore have three sides: we can discard (a) and (b).

2. Repeating the same process again, we're left with the inner and smaller shape, which most likely follows a similar sequence configuration; indeed, the smaller shape loses a side as it goes from a square to an upside down triangle. Applying this to the second statement, which has a small diamond with four sides, the inner shape in the second box should therefore have three sides.

The correct answer is (d). You'll get five of these sets in a row in the exam.

Type 4 Sets

Approach

Type 4 sets are essentially the same as Type 1 sets except you're asked to choose the test shape out of a selection of four that belongs to either Set A or Set B. You'll get five of these questions in a row for the same set. The approach and aim for Type 4 sets is the same - that is to locate a pattern.

The approach for these sets is exactly the same as for Type 1 sets:

1. Glance for any **obvious patterns**
2. **Compare** the two simplest and most similar boxes using SSSPN
3. **Confirm** in other boxes
4. **Apply** the pattern to the questions

Walkthrough

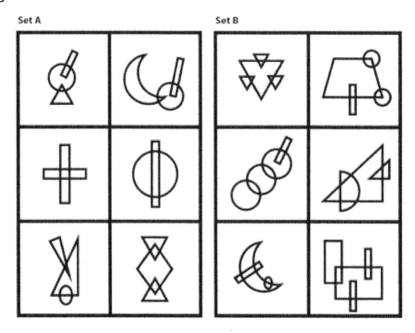

You should approach these sets the same way you would for a Type 1 set.

1. Glancing for any obvious patterns, we note intersecting objects: this is a common UCAT pattern, whereby either the number of intersections or number of enclosed areas are the same for each box in a set.

2. If we pick any box in Set A and counted, we find four intersections - this is our pattern. Similarly, there are six intersections in every box in Set B.

3. For the majority of questions, you'll have to go through the whole approach (comparing two simple boxes, SSSPN, etc.), but for a few questions, for example where you see intersections or arrows, the pattern will be much more obvious.

4. Once we have the pattern, we apply it to our questions.

1. Which of these belongs to Set A?

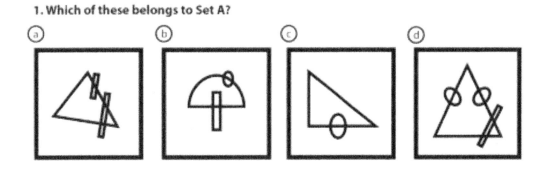

For the first Type 4 question, we're asked 'which of the following belongs to Set A?'.

Applying the pattern, we found to each of the four test shapes and counting the number of intersections in each test box, we find that (b) contains four intersections, which matches Set A. Continuing to the next question, which asks for the test shape that belongs to Set B, we find (b) is the correct answer because it has six intersections. The answers to the subsequent questions are (b) (belonging to Set A), (b) (belongs to Set B), and (d) (belonging to Set A).

Now try these...

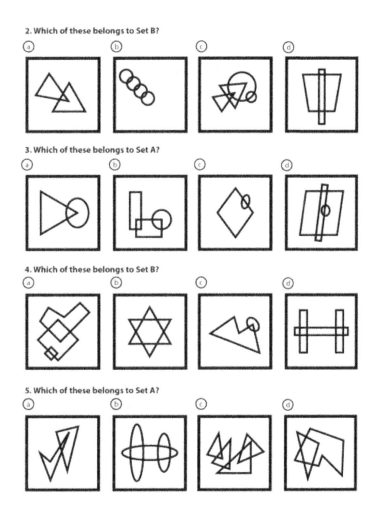

Complex Patterns

Dependent Patterns

Dependent patterns are where two pattern characteristics (SSSPN) in a box rely or depend on one other. For example, if there is a triangle in a box, there will be an arrow pointing upwards and if there is no triangle in the box there will be an arrow pointing downwards. These dependent sets are amongst the hardest you'll come across in AR - and although they do vary in difficulty, they tend to be the ones students most often get wrong. They are difficult because the patterns aren't always obvious and easy to tease out - they're usually the 'eureka' questions where you had to think outside the box to get to the pattern.

For this reason, you really should master the basic patterns if you want to have both the time and familiarity with common characteristics required to answer these questions. You must be able to work through SSSPN so that you can rule out any basic patterns, leaving some time to try out different combinations of characteristics that could yield a dependent pattern. Most dependent patterns simply connect together two simple patterns categories: for example, 'number' and 'shade' - if there are an odd number of shapes in the box, the diamond will be shaded black.

A lot of finding dependent patterns boils down to trial and error, but it is possible to narrow it down through discarding pattern categories (all shapes are the same 'shade' and 'size', or there are no obvious 'position' arrangements within a box). Don't feel too bad if you don't identify particularly difficult dependent patterns - most students don't, and most of your marks come from getting the basic questions right.

Walkthrough

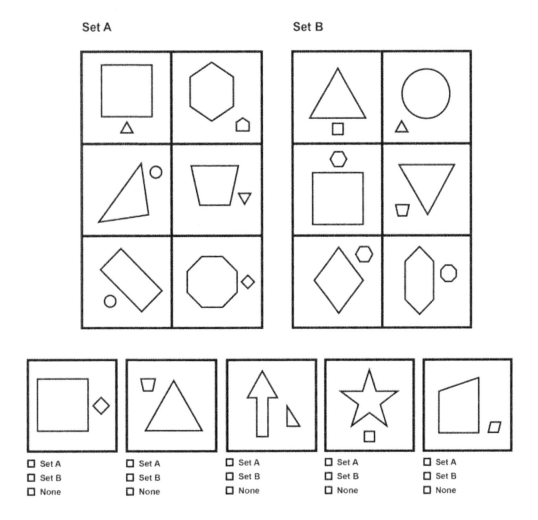

Set A   Set B

Running through SSSPN, we should focus on discarding categories that are probably irrelevant: there are no obvious shape patterns, and we can definitely discard shade. We should bear position in mind, although it's difficult to see any basic position pattern here.

As soon as we see this question, it's obvious that the differing sizes of the two shapes in each box plays a part of the pattern: there is always a big shape and a small shape, but that in itself isn't enough for the pattern because both Set A and Set B have big and small shapes, as well as all of the test boxes. We need to therefore find out what determines whether a shape is big or small.

Finding a more difficult pattern within a set can be harder, especially when it's more subtle: given the complementary nature of patterns between Set A and Set B, it may be helpful comparing the most similar two boxes from Set A and Set B. As we choose to go with the top left box from Set A (containing a large square and a small triangle), we find that there is a similar combination of shapes in the top left box from Set B, but instead with the triangle being bigger than the square. Comparing these two boxes, the only real modifying characteristic based upon basic patterns left (we've already discarded shape and shade), is the number of sides of a given shape affecting the size of the shape itself. Indeed, the square is bigger in Set A because it has more sides than the triangle, and vice versa for Set B.

The pattern is therefore

Set A - The bigger shape always has more sides than the smaller shape.

Set B - The bigger shape always has fewer sides than the smaller shape.

Answers:

Shape 1: None (the shapes have an equal number of sides)

Shape 2: Set B

Shape 3: Set A

Shape 4: Set A

Shape 5: None

Multi-Patterns

On the harder end of the spectrum for AR questions, there will be more than one pattern in a set. For example, Set A may have a circle in every box, but also four shapes, and an arrow always pointing upwards. These sets, as you probably realise, are time-consuming, and so it's important not to get held back and stubbornly continue looking for more patterns when your time has passed.

The problem is, it can be difficult to tell whether or not a set has multiple patterns. In general, sets that contain multiple patterns tend to be more complicated, with more objects. After finding one pattern, you must keep in mind that there may be something more going on. Of course, in reality, you won't know if you've missed any further patterns. The good news is that even if you've only identified two out of four patterns, the chances are you'll still get some marks if you apply them correctly to the test shapes. This doesn't mean that you should always wait around looking for more patterns, but you shouldn't move on too quickly in situations where you have some time left to do a seemingly complicated set.

Practice Questions

Unlike the other sets of practice questions - we can't really do this as a mock test because given the distribution of questions you'd get loads of practice of Type 1 and then you'd only have one of type 2, 3, or 4 included - which would be a bit rubbish if that wasn't the type which came up in the test.

So instead, we've included 10 Type 2 questions - which we recommend you try and do in 11 minutes (if you're working under timed conditions) - and then you can pick any one of the type 2, 3 or 4 sets to tag onto the end (if you're trying to do a full test). And treat the other two as practice!

1. For each of the shapes below, decide whether they belong to Set A, Set B or None.

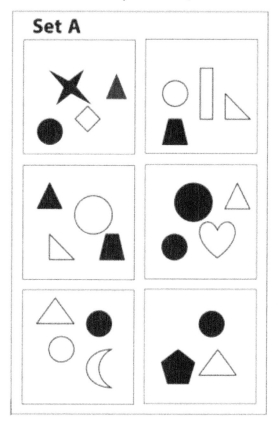 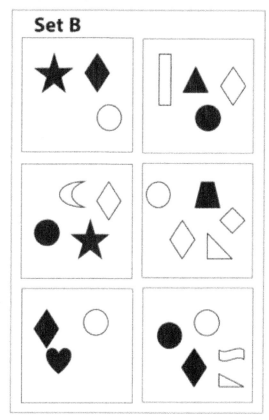

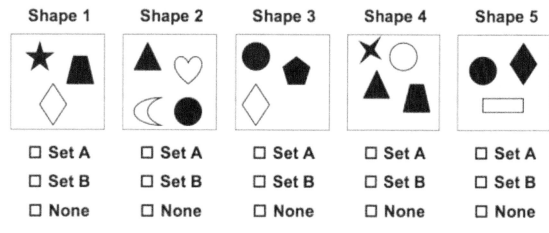

2. For each of the shapes below, decide whether they belong to Set A, Set B or None.

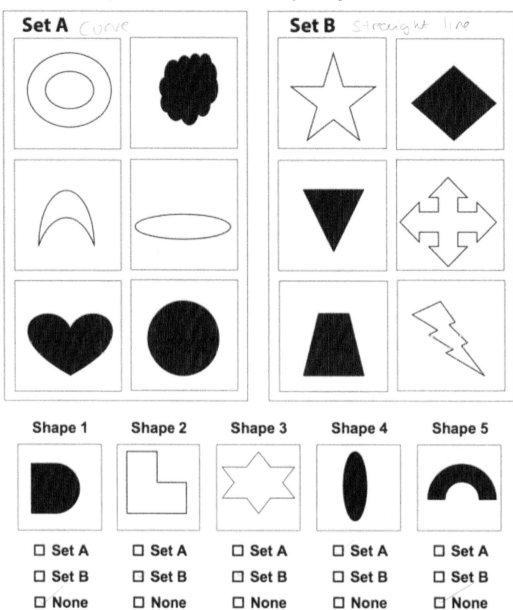

Shape 1	Shape 2	Shape 3	Shape 4	Shape 5
☐ Set A	☐ Set A	☐ Set A	☐ Set A	☐ Set A
☐ Set B	☐ Set B	☐ Set B	☐ Set B	☐ Set B
☐ None	☐ None	☐ None	☐ None	☐ None

3. For each of the shapes below, decide whether they belong to Set A, Set B or None.

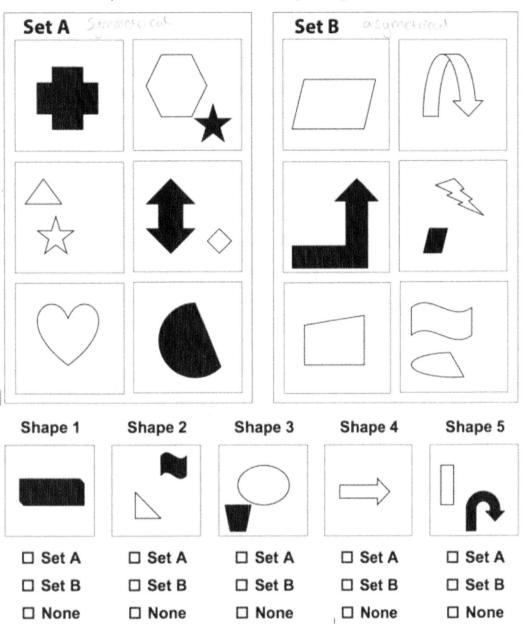

Shape 1

☐ Set A
☐ Set B
☐ None

Shape 2

☐ Set A
☐ Set B
☐ None

Shape 3

☐ Set A
☐ Set B
☐ None

Shape 4

☐ Set A
☐ Set B
☐ None

Shape 5

☐ Set A
☐ Set B
☐ None

4. For each of the shapes below, decide whether they belong to Set A, Set B or None.

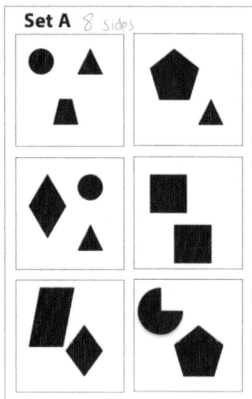

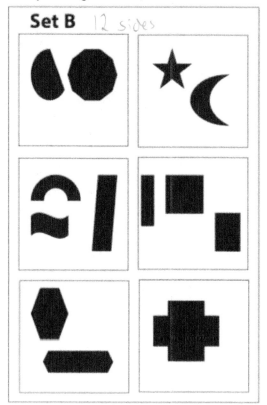

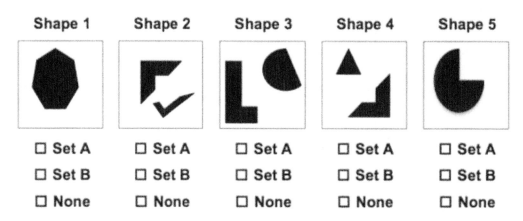

	Shape 1	Shape 2	Shape 3	Shape 4	Shape 5
	☐ Set A	☐ Set A	☐ Set A	☐ Set A	☐ Set A
	☐ Set B	☐ Set B	☐ Set B	☐ Set B	☐ Set B
	☐ None	☐ None	☐ None	☐ None	☐ None

5. For each of the shapes below, decide whether they belong to Set A, Set B or None.

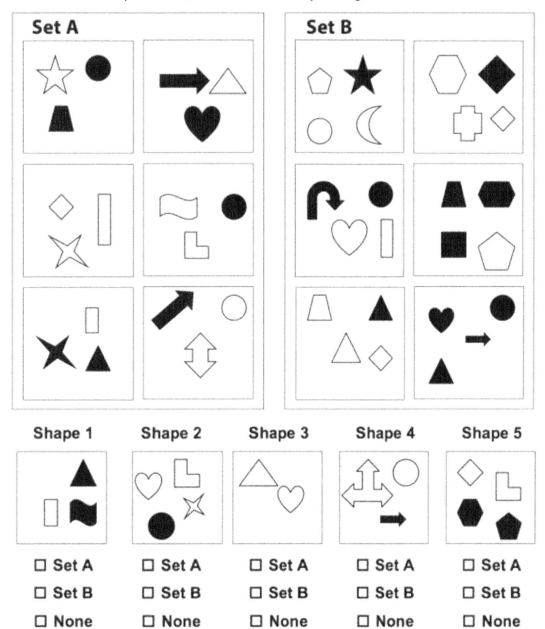

Shape 1	Shape 2	Shape 3	Shape 4	Shape 5
☐ Set A	☐ Set A	☐ Set A	☐ Set A	☐ Set A
☐ Set B	☐ Set B	☐ Set B	☐ Set B	☐ Set B
☐ None	☐ None	☐ None	☐ None	☐ None

6. For each of the shapes below, decide whether they belong to Set A, Set B or None.

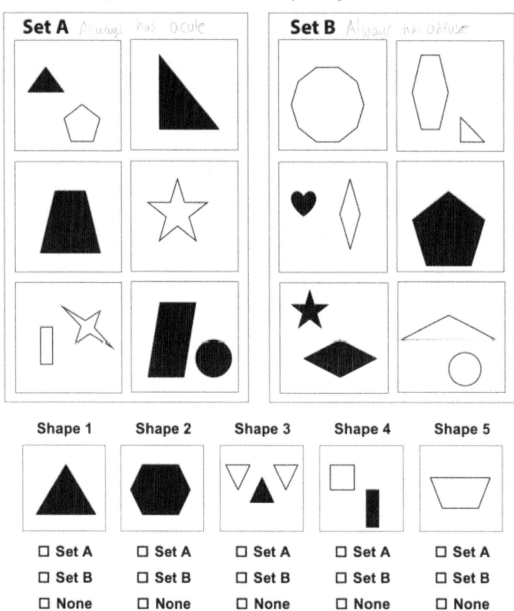

Set A *Always has acute*

Set B *Always has obtuse*

Shape 1	Shape 2	Shape 3	Shape 4	Shape 5
☐ Set A	☐ Set A	☐ Set A	☐ Set A	☐ Set A
☐ Set B	☐ Set B	☐ Set B	☐ Set B	☐ Set B
☐ None	☐ None	☐ None	☐ None	☐ None

7. For each of the shapes below, decide whether they belong to Set A, Set B or None.

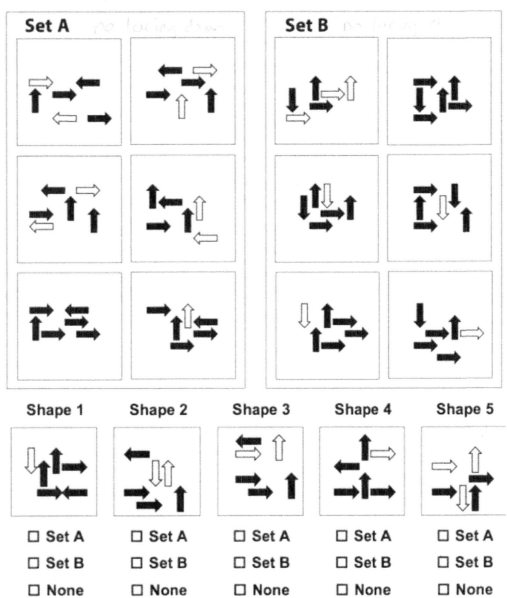

Shape 1	Shape 2	Shape 3	Shape 4	Shape 5
☐ Set A	☐ Set A	☐ Set A	☐ Set A	☐ Set A
☐ Set B	☐ Set B	☐ Set B	☐ Set B	☐ Set B
☐ None	☐ None	☐ None	☐ None	☐ None

8. For each of the shapes below, decide whether they belong to Set A, Set B or None.

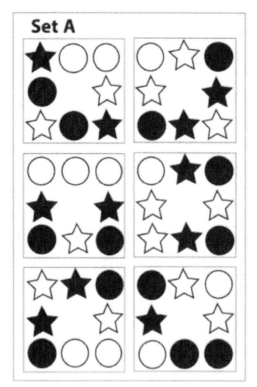 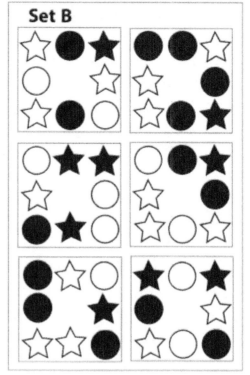

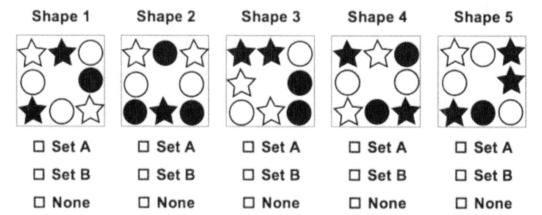

Shape 1	Shape 2	Shape 3	Shape 4	Shape 5
☐ Set A	☐ Set A	☐ Set A	☐ Set A	☐ Set A
☐ Set B	☐ Set B	☐ Set B	☐ Set B	☐ Set B
☐ None	☐ None	☐ None	☐ None	☐ None

9. For each of the shapes below, decide whether they belong to Set A, Set B or None.

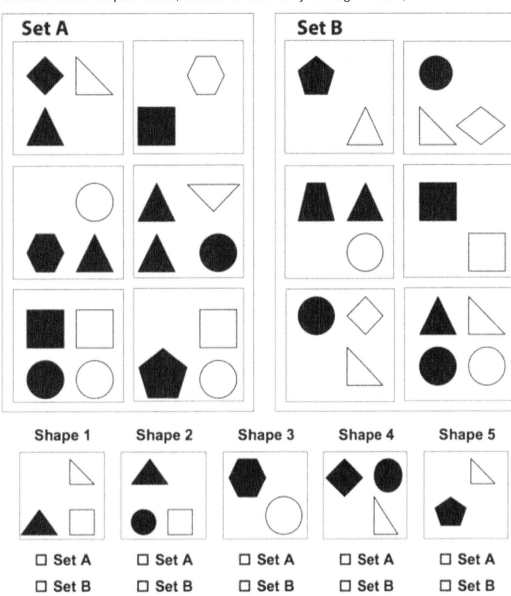

	Shape 1	Shape 2	Shape 3	Shape 4	Shape 5
Set A	☐	☐	☐	☐	☐
Set B	☐	☐	☐	☐	☐
None	☐	☐	☐	☐	☐

10. For each of the shapes below, decide whether they belong to Set A, Set B or None.

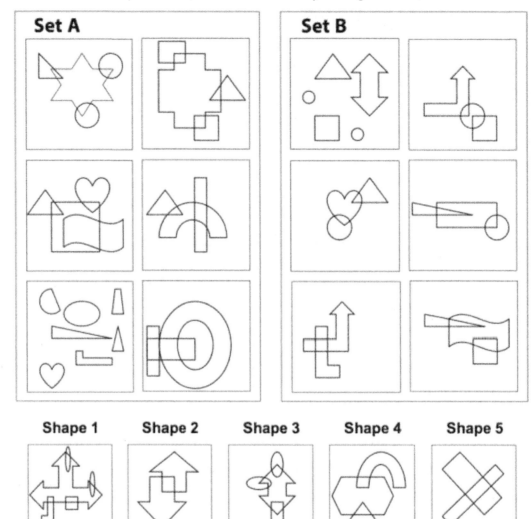

Shape 1	Shape 2	Shape 3	Shape 4	Shape 5
□ Set A	□ Set A	□ Set A	□ Set A	□ Set A
□ Set B	□ Set B	□ Set B	□ Set B	□ Set B
□ None	□ None	□ None	□ None	□ None

(Moving onto Type 2 sets!)

1. Is A, B, C or D the next shape in the series?

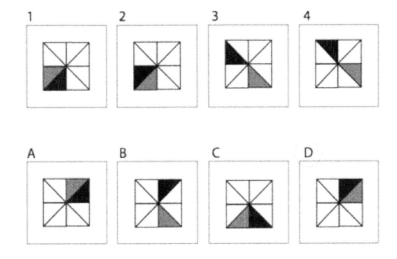

2. Is A, B, C or D the next shape in the series?

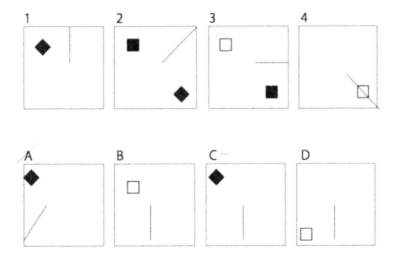

3. Is A, B, C or D the next shape in the series?

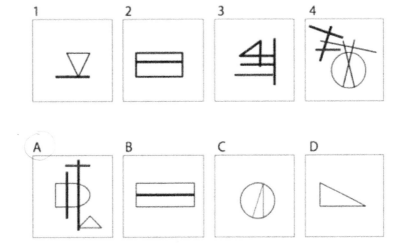

4. Is A, B, C or D the next shape in the series?

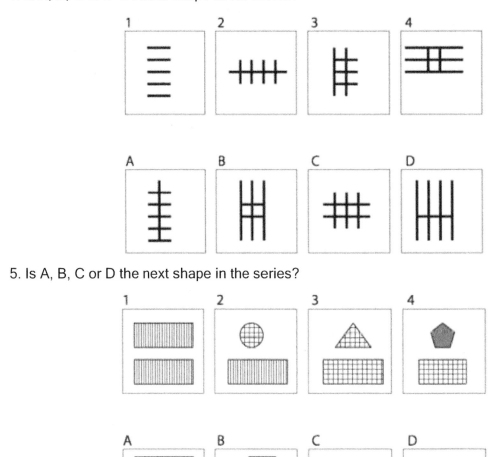

5. Is A, B, C or D the next shape in the series?

(Type 3! If you did the previous question in exam conditions you can stop here).

1. Is A, B, C or D the next shape in the series?

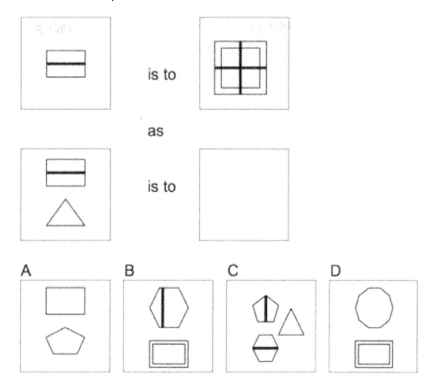

2. Is A, B, C or D the next shape in the series?

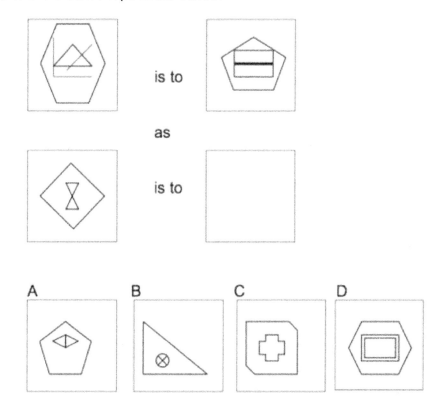

3. Is A, B, C or D the next shape in the series?

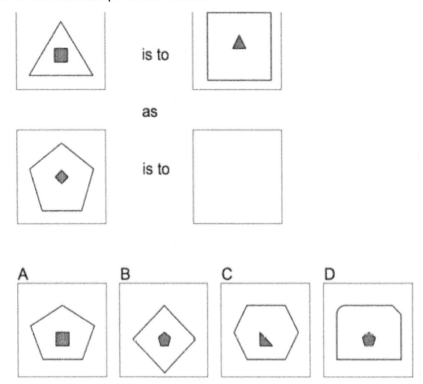

4. Is A, B, C or D the next shape in the series?

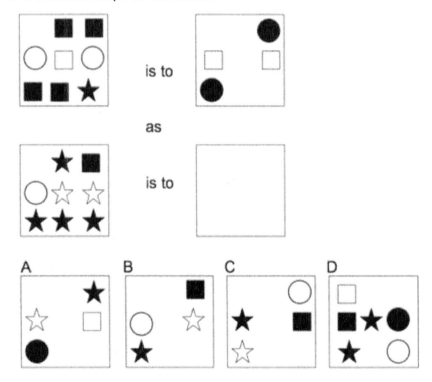

5. Is A, B, C or D the next shape in the series?

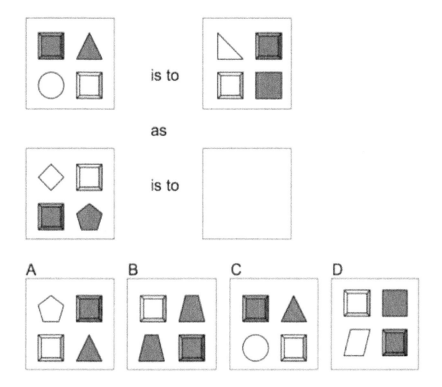

And finally – type 4! In the test you'd get 5 questions for each of these – but by now you've done so much Type 1 practice that it should be pretty quick!

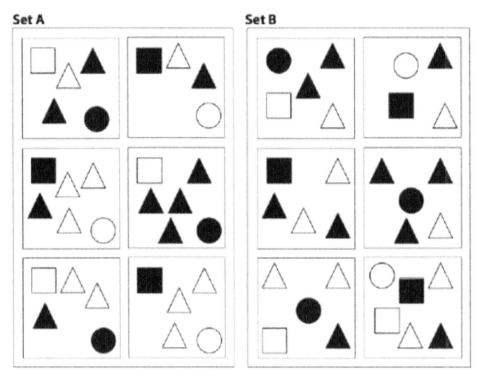

1. Which of the following shapes belong to Set A?

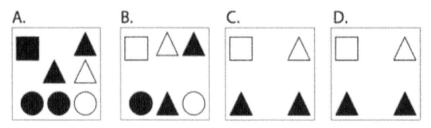

2. Which of the following shapes belong to Set B?

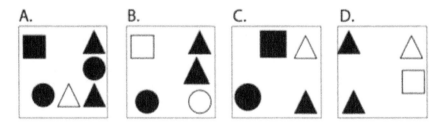

Solutions

Type One

<u>Set 1</u>

Group: Shape

Pattern:

Set A - Circle and triangle in every box

Set B - Diamond and circle in every box

Strategy: Running through SSSPN and comparing any two simple boxes in set A, we immediately see that there is a repeated circle, as well as a triangle. Indeed, upon checking other boxes, there is a circle and triangle in every box. It is reasonable to think that there may be other patterns, but it is evident there isn't a size pattern. We can also discard basic shading, position and number patterns. Thus, it is likely that the only pattern is a repeating circle and triangle in Set A. Similarly, we find a repeating diamond and circle in set B.

Answers:

Shape 1: None

Shape 2: Set A

Shape 3: Set B

Shape 4: Set A

Shape 5: Set B

<u>Set 2</u>

Group: Shape

Pattern:

Set A - Shapes are made up of only curved lines.

Set B - Shapes are made up of only straight lines.

Strategy: This is a relatively simple question, with each box containing only one shape. It should be immediately obvious what the pattern is: set A contains only curved lines, whereas set B contains only straight lines. Don't think that these patterns won't appear in the exam - they almost certainly do, and they are the ones which you must do as quickly as possible in order to leave more time elsewhere.

Answers:

Shape 1: None

Shape 2: Set B

Shape 3: Set B

Shape 4: Set A

Shape 5: None

Group: Symmetry

Pattern:

Set A - each box contains only symmetrical shapes

Set B - each box contains only asymmetrical shapes

Strategy: Each box is relatively simple, yet initially seems very different; however, closer examination reveals a shape pattern: each box in set a contains only symmetrical shapes, whereas set B boxes contain only asymmetrical shapes. Remember to compare two similar and simple boxes within a set, and then with the complementary set if need be. Just imagine taking a small mirror through each of the shapes.

Answers:

Shape 1: Set B

Shape 2: None

Shape 3: Set A

Shape 4: Sot A

Shape 5: None

Group: Number

Pattern:

Set A - total number of sides of shapes is 8.

Set B - total number of sides of shapes is 12.

Strategy: We can immediately discard most basic shape patterns - there is no clear repeating shape characteristic. Moreover, all the shapes are of a similar size and shading, as well as being positioned in an arbitrary manner. The only thing left is a potential number pattern, and it is clear that it isn't the number of shapes in each box. A common number pattern that is likely to make an appearance in the exam involves the total number of sides of all shapes in each box. Indeed, we can count 8 sides in each box in set A and 12 sides in set B.

Answers:

Shape 1: None

Shape 2: Set B

Shape 3: Set A

Shape 4: None

Shape 5: None

Group: Number pattern

Pattern:

Set A - each box contains 3 shapes

Set B - each box contains 4 shapes

Strategy: Comparing for a common shape characteristic between two boxes, we see that there is no immediately obvious repeating shape pattern. There aren't any obvious size, shading or position patterns either. The fact that there are 3 shapes in every box in set A and 4 shapes in every box in set B jumps out of the page - and this is indeed the pattern. This is another example of a question that can certainly come up and that should be done quickly without hesitation: it is easy to search

for further patterns, but the majority of questions are not difficult and can be represented by all the basic patterns and categories we've laid out. DON'T waste time looking for more patterns, and instead move on when you've discarded all basic patterns using SSSPN, unless the set looks seriously complicated and you have time to spare.

Answers:

Shape 1: Set A

Shape 2: Set B

Shape 3: None

Shape 4: Set A

Shape 5: Set B

Set 6

Group: Shape

Pattern:

Set A - every box contains at least one acute internal angle

Set B - every box contains at least one obtuse angle

Strategy: This question should only be more difficult if you haven't come across and noted down previous angle patterns. Nonetheless, the pattern may not be obvious even when comparing two simple boxes in set A, such as the right angle triangle and white star. There is clearly no basic size, shading, position or number pattern between these two shapes. It may be more helpful to compare the white star with the decagon in the top left box of set B: when stuck for patterns within a set, it is useful to contrast a simple box with another simple box in set B, which is usually complementary to set A.

Indeed, the only clear difference between the decagon and star (or right angle triangle in set A) is the presence of internal obtuse angles in the decagon and acute angles in the star. Further checking confirms that there is always at least one obtuse angle in each box in set B and an acute angle for each box in set A.

Answer:

Shape 1: Set A

Shape 2: Set B

Shape 3: Set A

Shape 4: None

Shape 5: None (both obtuse and acute angles present, meaning it could belong to either set A or set B hence answer is none).

Set 7

Group: Position

Pattern:

Set A - each box has arrows pointing in all directions except down. (No arrows pointing down)

Set B - each box has arrows pointing in all directions except left. (No arrows pointing left)

Strategy: When arrows are involved, there is a good chance that they are involved in a position pattern. In this set, we can eliminate a shading pattern, where it is inconsistent between boxes. Moreover, each box contains 6 arrows, with arbitrary numbers of arrows pointing towards any given direction across boxes. The only pattern that remains is represented by the direction the arrows are pointing, with each arrow in set A pointing towards every direction (up, right, left) except down. Similarly, in Set B, arrows point in every direction (up, right, down) except left.

Answers:

Shape 1: None

Shape 2: None

Shape 3: Set A

Shape 4: Set A

Shape 5: Set B

Set 8

Group: Position

Pattern:

Set A - the shading is now rearranged in a set order (an easy way of seeing it is by looking at the corner between two shaded shapes, it is always white, and also between two shaded shapes on a side - it is also always white.).

Set B - objects are all in the same rotational order (arranged relative to one another in a set order 2 stars, 2 circles, 1 star, 1 circle, 1 star, 1 circle)

Strategy: Immediately we notice a consistent, repeating arrangement of shapes and shading across all boxes, which allows us to discard a shape pattern, as well as size and number. Such repeating arrangements usually indicate a set position pattern. In this case, set A contains set relative shading positions and set B involves set relative shape positions. The easiest way to discern these patterns is through comparing two boxes and checking the pattern with further boxes.

Answers:

Shape 1: Set B

Shape 2: None

Shape 3: Set A

Shape 4: Set B

Shape 5: None

Set 9

Group: Position

Pattern:

Set A - there is a black shape in the bottom left corner and a white shape in the top right corner

Set B - there is a black shape in the top left corner and a white shape in the bottom right corner

Strategy: Comparing two simple boxes in set A, we find no basic shape pattern and the sizes of all shapes are roughly equal. There are both black and white shapes in set A and set B and variable numbers of shapes in each box. There is a black shape in the bottom left corner and a white shape in the top right corner, and this is consistent in all boxes in set A. Similarly, there is a black shape in the top left corner of each box in set B and a white shape in the bottom right corner.

Answers:

Shape 1: Set A

Shape 2: Set B

Shape 3: Set B

Shape 4: Set B

Shape 5: None

Set 10

Group: Number

Pattern:

Set A - there are 7 enclosed areas in each box

Set B - there are 5 enclosed areas in each box

Strategy: In this question, we can immediately see that shapes within each box are overlapping, forming intersections between lines and enclosed areas. A common UCAT question when it comes to overlapping shapes is either the number of intersections or enclosed areas. Because not all boxes contain overlapping shapes, we should consider a pattern involving enclosed areas. It is reasonable to put aside SSSPN initially and count for both these characteristics when coming across such a question: indeed, there are 7 enclosed areas in each box in set A and 5 enclosed areas in each box in set B.

Answers:

Shape 1: None

Shape 2: None

Shape 3: Set A

Shape 4: Set B

Shape 5: Set B

Type Two

1. Answer: D

Group: Position.

Sequence: Black is in a clockwise sequence. Grey is in an anti-clockwise sequence.

2. Answer: C

Group: Position.

Sequence: All shapes in the top left corner move to the bottom right corner in the subsequent box. Because there is no shape in the top left corner for the fourth box, it is assumed that the sequence will repeat itself. The line moves 45 degrees clockwise in each box.

3. Answer: A

Group: Number.

Sequence: In each box of the series, there is an increase of one line in each box.

4. Answer: D

Group: Number.

Sequence: There is an increase of one long line and a decrease of one short line, in each box.

5. Answer: C

Group: Shading.

Sequence: A new colour in the top shape in a box determines the shading of the subsequent box. (The bottom shape always remains as a rectangle.)

Type Three

1. Answer C

Group: Number.

Sequence: In each box, double the number of lines of the preceding box.

2. Answer: B

Group: Number.

Sequence: There is a descending sequence of both the number sides of the expanded shape, and the number of lines within the box. (The number of lines within the expanded shape matches the number of sides of the shape.)

3. Answer: B

Group: Size

Sequence: The larger shape becomes the smaller shape in the subsequent box, and the smaller shape of the preceding box becomes the expanded shape

4. Answer: A

Group: Position

Sequence: The bottom left shape has swapped positions with the one above it. The top right shape has swapped with the one below it. All swapped shapes have the taken on their opposite shading. The other shapes have all disappeared.

5. Answer: D

Group: Position & Shading.

Sequence: The two squares are in mirror positions in each subsequent box. The other shapes alternate shading.

Type Four

1. Answer: A

Group: Position & Shading

Pattern: In Set A, there is always a square in the top left corner, and a circle in the bottom right corner. If the square is white, the circle is black, and vice versa.

2. Answer: C

Group: Position & Shading

Pattern: In Set B, there is always a triangle in the bottom and top right hand corner. If the triangle in the bottom right corner is not shaded, the triangle in the top right corner is shaded, and vice versa.

Situational Judgement

What is 'Situational Judgement'?

The SJT gives you hypothetical scenarios and tests your judgement by asking how you would respond and examining why. These scenarios are medical or academic situations, in which you are generally a junior doctor, dentist or student. These tests have been around for years, and you'll find them used in a wide range of professions. They're useful because they assess non-academic, yet human qualities and can help determine practical intelligence in the workplace.

Why do we have to do the SJT?

As an applicant to medical school, you should be able to prove in the SJT that you can be competent in a hospital environment and deal with difficult situations in the right way. You'll be expected to display good ethical awareness and that you have interpersonal qualities that enable effective communication with colleagues and patients.

This won't be the last SJT exam you'll do - in the final year at medical school, students are required to take another SJT exam that plays a large part in applications to hospitals for FY1. Throughout your career, you will have to ensure you act appropriately and make the right decisions. You won't always have somebody looking over your shoulder, and when it comes down to it, you're working with people's lives - it isn't surprising that medical schools want to make sure you're not going to put patients at risk.

Numbers for this Section

When it comes to anything in the UCAT, getting to grips with the timing is essential - make sure you don't just know how much time you have, but understand how to practically apply time limits to your practice.

Here's a table on how much time you're given for SJT:

| 1 minute | Instructions |
| 26 minutes | 69 items (22 sets of 2-5 items each) |

If we break it down further, we get the following:

| ~ 20 seconds | Time per question |
| Q.35 with 13 minutes remaining | Halfway marker |

Question Types

You'll be given 22 scenarios; each relating to a dispute between what a doctor, dentist or student is supposed to be doing, and a problem that comes up in or outside of the workplace. This problem might involve difficult behaviour by a patient or colleague, or an external personal matter, making it hard to carry out normal tasks. Remember the all-important quality needed in a doctor - empathy - and try to put yourself "in the shoes" of the person responding to the situation. Each dilemma is followed by 2-5 questions, which are either 'appropriateness' or 'importance' questions.

The initial part of the section (approximately half to two-thirds of the questions) are 'appropriateness' questions, where you've got to figure out whether possible responses to the situation in the scenario are appropriate or inappropriate (on a scale of 1-4). The second part of the section (approximately one-third to half of the questions) are 'importance' questions, where you need to establish how important (again, on a scale of 1-4) various factors should be in determining your response.

Besides the general 'appropriateness' and 'importance' questions, there's also a new type of question added this year. Here you are given 3 possible actions to a scenario, and you have to choose which response is the 'most appropriate', and which response is the 'least appropriate'. This question is quite similar to the 'appropriateness' questions, however, requires some extra thought.

Instead of simply assessing the appropriateness of one action, you need to go through all 3 actions separately, and compare them to assess which one is the most or least appropriate action relative to the scenario. Since there are multiple actions to assess, this new type of question might take more time than the other situational judgement questions, and therefore it is important to be wary of time when doing these.

Unlike the previous sections, the SJT isn't scored on a scale of 300 to 900. Rather, you'll be assessed from Band 1 to Band 4: According to the UKCAT website, band 1 is 'exceptional performance', band 2 is 'good', band 3 is 'below average' and band 4 is 'poor'. The band reflects the extent to which your answers match the answers as agreed on by a panel of medical experts. Band 1 means that most of your answers were similar to the panel, whereas band 4 means that very few of your answers were similar - let's hope that's not the case! Therefore, the main aim of the SJT is to pick the same answer as the panel of clinical professionals. Even if, on a personal level, you may not respond in a particular way, if you're aware that something is more or less appropriate in the eyes of universities/medics/dentists, then go by "what is right".

Due to the fact that scoring is different to other sections (and this is a relatively new section), universities use the results differently to other sections of the UKCAT. For example, University of Birmingham has said that it considers SJT at the interview stage, whereas University of Nottingham gives each section, including SJT (albeit to a lesser extent), a score to decide which students to invite to interview. Please take this into account and be intelligent when applying to universities, as there's no point in applying to a university which has a cut-off at Band 2 if you yourself have sadly received a Band 3 in UKCAT.

But that's not going to happen...

Preparation Tips

Section Structure and Difficulties

Congratulations on making it to the final section! Most people think this section is the simplest of the UKCAT, based purely on natural instinct, but there is some skill to it you can pick up through preparation and practice. Although there is a lot of common sense in this section, you have to stay on the ball and ready to respond to the scenarios they throw at you. This can be difficult because you might be getting fatigued by this point in the exam. It's really easy to get complacent with time, but keep in mind how pressed for time you actually are (see table on the previous page). Your preparation for the SJT section can also be useful for your interview, especially if you read up on common ethical scenarios, and how they can be approached.

Competencies being tested

Interpersonal competencies

This is relevant for the SJT, personal statements, interviews, and life in general, so be sure to have a skim through these, even if you think you know/have every competency under the sun (humility might need working on if the latter's the case!) It refers to your ability as a doctor, dentist or medical student to build effective working relationships with colleagues, senior doctors and patients. This skillset involves:

1. **Decision making:** a doctor is entrusted with the responsibility of putting patient care first. Doing this requires making important decisions on a daily basis, often while under considerable pressure. As a doctor, you will need to take all relevant information into account, focusing on the most important aspects, when making these decisions. It is also your responsibility to flag up any issues if colleagues are not taking the same care with their decision making.

2. **Leadership:** to motivate and develop other members involved in the patient's care

3. **Communication (speaking and listening):** strong communicators make good team members because they can efficiently and effectively transfer critical information. In medicine, this may

involve reporting a patient's history, following instructions that have been given to you and instructing others.

4. Teamwork: doctors cannot function alone. You must get on with other medical professionals and work with them efficiently and effectively. Members of the team could include: doctors (GPs, physicians, surgeons), nurses, pharmacists, radiologists, dieticians, hospital attendants, managerial staff, and, most importantly, the patient!

5. Empathy: you must respond appropriately to the patient's concerns and treat people with dignity and respect at all times.

6. Humility: it is important not to allow knowledge or power to inflate your ego. Acting out of arrogance is not admirable and will not secure you a good score in the UCAT.

7. Dealing with authority: as a doctor or medical student, it will be a while before you make it to the top of your profession. You'll need to respect senior doctors and experts, and learn from their knowledge and experience as much as possible.

Ethical competencies

Ethics can be defined as "dealing with values relating to human conduct and philosophy." It takes into account the right and wrong of actions and their underlying rationales. Medical ethics therefore deals with the values and guidelines governing decision-making in medical practice. Some are written codes, which state the ethical guidelines a doctor must consider when performing their duties, and others are unwritten truths. Ethical conduct is highly important for a doctor as you will encounter such dilemmas concerning human lives on a daily basis.

The most important principles in medical ethics include: staying motivated to give effective medical care, maintaining professional standards, safeguarding patient confidentiality within the constraints of the law, following duty of candour (make patients aware of all relevant information), and striving to learn, apply, and progress scientific knowledge.

The ethical competencies tested in this section are based on the guidelines laid out by the GMC in their 'Good Medical Practice' handbook. This handbook, which should be read by all doctors, outlines the key principles of medical professionalism in a way that is directly applicable to scenarios that doctors come across every day. We advise you to have a read through this document, a PDF of which can be found on google, to familiarise yourself with the principles that are valued the GMC and therefore most likely to be tested in the UCAT.

You can get a copy of the GMC Good Medical Practice by such searching on google and heading over to the GMCs website.

Strategy

The Holistic Method

1. Always **read the scenario** before readying the first question. It is impossible to start thinking about the appropriateness of responses or importance of factors before you have gotten to grips with the situation. It may be tempting to skim read the scenarios to save time, as you have been doing for VR and maybe even QR, but this is not advisable for the situational judgement section. If you skim read, you might overlook vital information that could drastically change your response to a scenario. Reading the scenario probably takes around 30 seconds, but this may improve as you practise speed reading for the verbal section and become more familiar with the types of scenario that typically come up. Remember, once you've read the scenario once, it can be quickly glossed over to refresh your memory if necessary when it comes to answering the questions.

2. As you **read the responses**, make it second nature to rapidly **pick a side**. Is the response appropriate or inappropriate? Is the factor important or not? This will help you to narrow down the options from four to two. You can then think about whether the extreme option or the intermediate option is correct, but regardless you are awarded partial marks for coming down on the right side.

3. **Decide when to choose the intermediate options.** In the rest of the exam, there is an equal likelihood of any answer option being correct - but this is not true of the SJT! Some UCAT-loving statisticians analysed the UCAT's official practice materials and found something very interesting. They showed that the answers are weighted at the extremes (e.g. very appropriate, very inappropriate, very important and not important at all), with the intermediate answers (appropriate but not ideal, inappropriate but not awful, important and of minor importance) only being right about 30% of the time.

With this in mind, it's still OK to choose the intermediate options when the response is less than optimal for some reason, or when the possible negative consequences of that response are not severe. We will explore this in more detail in the sections below.

Important Points

A few things that are worth considering when following the 6med strategy:

1. **Not every set of items has one of each answer.**

This is a classic mistake made by students. It could very well be the case that there are no 'inappropriate, but not awful' answers; equally it could very well be that all of the answers are 'very inappropriate'

2. **Medical and dental students are not yet fully-fledged clinicians.**

Remember, you must always behave within the **limits of your competence** and look for help if you're being asked to do something beyond your remit. For example, if there is a scenario in which a patient is asking a medical student about their test results, it wouldn't be appropriate for the student to make a diagnosis. This is because the student may not yet be equipped with the medical knowledge required to do this and because the doctor may have planned how to break the bad news.

3. Core principles such as **confidentiality**, **consent** and **patient safety** will come up, so be sure to look into them before sitting the UKCAT. Social media in particular (Facebook, Twitter, YouTube) is a new challenge to medicine, notorious for breaching confidentiality and compromising professionalism. Remember too that ensuring your own wellbeing as a practising provider of healthcare is important in order to provide optimal care.

4.. Last and definitely not least, a situation is likely to mention multiple characters - make sure you are aware of the person who is supposed to be responding as this can alter the outcome drastically.

Appropriateness

Definitions

Taken from the UCAT website, here are the options you'll be dealing with and what they mean:

- a **very appropriate** thing to do if it will address at least one aspect (not necessarily all aspects) of the situation

- **appropriate**, but not ideal if it could be done, but is not necessarily a very good thing to do

- **inappropriate**, but not awful if it should not really be done, but would not be terrible

- a **very inappropriate** thing to do if it should definitely not be done and would make the situation worse

Important Points

- **Never** judge a response as though it's the only thing that is done.

  For example, in hospital, if the wrong medication is has given to a patient, there are multiple steps that should be taken. This means that there are multiple 'very appropriate' responses that should all be carried out. In this example, asking the patient how they feel and assessing them medically are both 'very appropriate' responses. Remember, the responses should not be judged as if they are the only action taken. Many students would read these two options (asking the patient how they feel and assessing them medically) and assume that one must be 'very appropriate' and the other 'appropriate but not ideal' - but this is simply not how the exam works. Having said this, if two responses are very similar, you should think about what one may be lacking. This response may be 'appropriate but not ideal'.

- As providers of high quality healthcare, we shouldn't just deal with the symptoms, but should look for the underlying pathology.
  - Similarly, when dealing with difficult situations, it's important to try to get to the **root of the problem** rather than alleviating just one of the outcomes

- **Natural intellect** (good old common sense!) always comes in handy when picking a side, and it is usually right. So don't restrict that gut instinct from telling you what it thinks.

- Remember that the **patient's needs should always be put first**.

  For example, if patient is anxious, it would be inappropriate for the doctor to simply dismiss the patient. As this would make matters worse, rather than just not make it better, this response is 'very inappropriate' rather than 'inappropriate but not awful'. Similarly, it would be unprofessional to break patient-doctor trust by asking another doctor to console your patient. Therefore, this would also be a 'very inappropriate' response.

- When there is an issue that needs more senior involvement, it is **important to escalate appropriately**.

  A response that involves reporting an issue to someone much more senior tends to be on the 'inappropriate' side of the spectrum. This is because it is important not to blow things out of proportion and it is best to resolve minor issues at a local level. The main exception to this is when patient safety is at risk and the only way to solve the issue is by going to a consultant.

- Finally, remember that dignity and respect are key within the workplace. Automatically go for the inappropriate side of the scale if colleagues or patients are being treated unfairly or rudely.

The Holy Trinity

The Holy Trinity describes the three key qualities of a 'very appropriate' response. Once you've cracked this, you should be able to appreciate that if a response has some, but not all, of these qualities then it will be 'appropriate but not ideal'. If it shows few or none of these qualities, then it will be 'inappropriate but not awful' and if it **makes it worse**, it will be 'very inappropriate'.

The Holy Trinity of SJT appropriateness success:
1. Effective
2. Well-timed
3. Professional

First andforemost, an appropriate response must effectively address at least one element of the problem at hand. Secondly, an appropriate response must be well-timed. This usually means responding rapidly, but sometimes it is more appropriate to wait e.g. until the end of a patient consultation, as interrupting may undermine the doctor.

Professionalism encompasses many things, including respecting confidentiality, treating patients and colleagues fairly and responding tactfully. For example, shouting at a colleague who looks distracted during a procedure in front of the patient is unprofessional, taking them to a separate room to remind them of what is required for good medical practice would be preferred. Unprofessional actions include anything that may put patient safety at risk, acting outside of the limits of your competency, failing to escalate issues appropriately and getting involved in inappropriate relationships with patients.

Usually, when the response is merely a lack of action, it is considered 'inappropriate but not awful'. However, when this lack of action makes matters worse, e.g. failing to stop a conversation where confidentiality is being breached, then it is considered 'very inappropriate'.

Walkthrough

Here's a quick worked example to get a feel for the sort of question you'll be asked:

Roger is a medical student accompanying two junior doctors Mark and Amy. The two junior doctors are making fun of one of the patients on the ward. The patient is within earshot and looks visibly distressed but doesn't say anything.

How appropriate are each of the following responses by Roger in this situation?

1. Quietly mention to the junior doctors that the patient can hear them and is looking uneasy.

> **Very appropriate** – subtle and delicate, deals with the problem at once, and stops the patient losing faith in medical professionals.

2. At the end of the day mention to the junior doctors that their behaviour was inappropriate.

> **Appropriate but not ideal** – doesn't deal with the problem rapidly at the point at which the issue is occurring.

3. Tell Mark and Amy's overseeing senior consultant about their behaviour at the end of the week.

> **Very inappropriate** – isn't subtle/delicate, nor does it deal with the problem at the time and blows the whole situation out of proportion when it could have been resolved locally.

4. Audibly lecture Mark and Amy about how unprofessional and upsetting their behaviour is.

> **Very inappropriate** – lacks professionalism, patient may lose faith in Roger too, and it isn't subtle/delicate.

5. Apologize to the patient on behalf of Mark and Amy later that day.

> **Very inappropriate** – patient is guaranteed to lose faith in Mark and Amy as they haven't apologized themselves. Furthermore, they have not been made aware of their wrongdoing so could continue to do so in the future, making matters worse.

Importance

Definitions

You'll be asked how important various considerations are to take into account when deciding how to respond to the situation. The options (as taken from the UCAT website) are: very important if this is something that is vital to take into account

1. important if this is something that is important but not vital to take into account
2. of minor importance if this is something that could be taken into account, but it does not matter if it is considered or not
3. not important at all if this is something that should definitely not be taken into account

Read these carefully, especially the one for 'not important at all' because it is easy to think of something that is quite irrelevant as 'not important at all' when in fact it wouldn't matter if it was taken into account, so should therefore be 'of minor importance'.

Important Points

In a similar fashion to our approach to appropriateness questions, 6med has devised a trinitarian formula for responding to importance questions:

1. Ensure the aspect to be considered is relevant to the situation
2. Put those under your care first (4 key medical ethics)
3. Follow the rules of the workplace

Importance' scenarios are usually malpractice situations, and remember that you must consider the factors independently of each other, so all answers could be very important, or not important at all. Something that you should also remember: if something could be deemed generally 'very important' in most situations, it may not actually be relevant to the specific course of action that is being taken for a certain scenario. In other words, it all depends on the situation - don't make assumptions, because context is important.

As medical professionals, your first priority is those under your care (patients and juniors).

You must always follow the rules and guidelines, and adhere to the expectations of your workplace. Clinical guidelines have been put in place to protect patients, professionals and the public, and to ensure a standardised approach to effective clinical practice and safe patient care. Thus, this consideration is always very important. Malpractice (such as breaching confidentiality) must always be addressed, even if the perpetrator had good intentions, e.g. sharing patient information for education. Also, on a side note, you're applying to a medical/dental school guys and girls, so obviously they don't want rule-breakers.

Here are some selected requirements set out in the UCL Medical School Code of Conduct, we've emboldened the stuff that the SJT tests:

- **You are expected to listen to patients and respect their views, treat them politely considerately, respect patients' privacy and dignity and respect their right to refuse to take part in teaching.**

- You should not allow personal views about a person's age, disability, lifestyle, culture, beliefs, ethnic or national origin, race, colour, gender, sexual orientation, marital or parental status, social or perceived economic status to **prejudice** your interaction with patients, teachers, professional services staff or colleagues.

- You are expected to be honest. You should not abuse the trust of a patient or other vulnerable person. **You should not plagiarize** material from other sources and submit it as your own work. **Dishonesty is a fitness to practice issue**.

- You should not enter into an **improper personal relationship** with another person, for example, with a school pupil whom you are mentoring or a member of staff who is teaching you.

- You must always make clear to patients that you are a student and not a qualified doctor. Introducing yourself as a "medical student" or "training to be a doctor" is preferable to describing yourself as a "student doctor". You must always act within the direction of your educational supervisor(s) and **within the remit and competencies of a medical student.**

- You are bound by the **principle of confidentiality** of patient records and patient data. You must therefore take all reasonable precautions to ensure that any personal data relating to patients that you have learned by virtue of your position as a medical student will be kept confidential.

- You should not discuss patients with other students or professionals outside the clinical setting, except anonymously. When recording data or discussing cases outside the clinical setting you must endeavour to ensure that patients cannot be identified by others. You must respect all hospital and practice patient records.

- You are expected to maintain appropriate standards of dress, appearance, and personal hygiene so as not to cause offence to patients, teachers, or colleagues. The appearance of a student should not be such as to potentially affect a patient's confidence in their professional standing.

- You are expected to be aware of **safe drinking guidelines for alcohol** and to adhere to these guidelines. Misuse of alcohol and **any use of an illegal drug is a fitness to practice issue.**

- You are required physically to examine patients of both sexes (which includes touching and intimate examinations) in order to establish a clinical diagnosis, irrespective of the gender, culture, beliefs, disability, or

- disease of the patient. In order to qualify as a doctor in the UK, it is required that the practitioner is willing to examine any patient as fully and as intimately as is clinically necessary.

- You are required to keep your health clearance and immunizations up-to-date and to inform the Divisional Tutor of any changes which might affect your ability to undertake Exposure Prone Procedures (EPPs), e.g. exposure to, or infection with, blood-borne viruses.

- You must **inform** us if you are investigated, charged with, or convicted of a criminal offence during your time as a student at UCL Medical School.

- You must inform us if there is any significant change to your health that might affect your fitness to study medicine or to practice as a doctor.

Walkthrough

Here's a quick worked example to get a feel for the sorts of question you'll be asked:

Joe, a final year medical student, comes to the ward extremely hung-over and complains to Anna that he hasn't slept all night and still feels drunk. Joe mentions that this is the third time this month that this has happened and that he really should stop. He also recounts to Anna that he's found it difficult to carry out examinations when he's previously been in this state.

How important to take into account are the following considerations for Anna when deciding how to respond to the situation?

1. Joe has been asked to carry out a difficult procedure today

> **Very important** – being hungover/drunk on the ward impairs clinical judgement, compromises skill in practical procedures and reduces public confidence in healthcare professionals. Therefore, even if Joe hadn't been asked to perfom a difficult procedure today, we should be concerned by this unprofessional behaviour. However, this factor is still very important because it increases the urgency with which we must respond. Joe certainly shouldn't be carrying out any difficult procedures in his current state, so Anna must respond rapidly to ensure that patient safety is not compromised.

2. The medical school issued strict rules at the start of the year prohibiting students from being under the influence of alcohol/illegal drugs whilst on duty

> **Very Important**– it's important to follow rules and guidelines, especially as a medical professional.

3. Several other students are in a similar state to Joe

> **Of minor importance** – the fact that others are in a similar state to Joe doesn't excuse unprofessional and potentially dangerous behaviour. This factor should not necessarily influence how Anna should respond to the issue at hand and therefore does not come down on the 'important' side of things. However, it wouldn't matter if it were taken into account, because informing a higher-up as to the full extent of the situation could lead to systematic changes to prevent this from happening.

4. Joe has made a bet with another student this morning that he won't be disciplined for being in this state

> **Not important at all** – this bet is immature and unprofessional but should not influence Anna's response.

5. Keeping the information Joe has disclosed between them to maintain confidentiality

> **Not important at all** – the patient is of primary concern, so we must tell someone higher up, especially as this is a repeated offence. Joe's confidentiality therefore definitely shouldn't be taken into account.

Practice Questions

The SJT is quite a long section in the UCAT - so rather than including an entire practice test we'd suggest you do your practice tests under timed conditions on the UCAT website or ukcat.ninja after you've used these as practice.

Set 1

Adele is a nurse who suddenly approaches Dr. Liam as the patient she has been treating wishes to see a doctor. The patient complains to Dr. Liam of Adele's immaturity and poor bedside manner. The patient is evidently annoyed at having been made to wait a very long time.

How appropriate are each of the following responses by Dr. Liam in this situation?

A. Clarify with the patient in what way Adele has been immature.

B. Clarify with the nurse after the consultation how she felt it went.

C. Apologise for making the patient wait a long time.

D. Tell Adele to apologise immediately.

E. Apologise for Adele's poor bedside manner and immaturity.

Set 2

Parth, a medical student, is talking to a patient, Luma, at a General Practice. He has been given her notes by the GP, Dr Morris. Luma confides in Parth about how she is anxious about a new course of steroids she is being prescribed; however, Parth has been told by Dr Morris that the patient's medication is not being changed.

How appropriate are each of the following responses by Parth in this situation?

A. He asks Luma why she is worried.

B. He encourages Luma to voice her concerns to the GP.

C. He tells Dr Morris the patient's concerns.

D. He tells Luma she has nothing to worry about.

E. He opens up Luma's records of past history and examinations to check past medications.

Set 3

Melissa the secretary notices the smell of alcohol on Dr. George's breath, and patients have been complaining about his mistakes since yesterday. She is aware that he recently suffered the loss of his mother and fears he may not be dealing with it too well. She informs the other GP at the practice, Dr. Fred, about her concerns.

How appropriate are each of the following responses by Dr. Fred in this situation?

A. Report Dr. George to the GMC for his unprofessional attitude.

B. Stay out of the situation and encourage the receptionist to air her own concerns with Dr George.

C. Talk delicately with Dr. George recommending he take some more time off.

D. Tell the receptionist that he spoke with Dr. George yesterday and reassure her that all is well, when in actual fact his conversation with Dr. George was just in passing.

E. Look into the recent complaints that have been made to help ascertain Dr. George's behaviour.

Set 4

Homer and Lesley have recently started their clinical attachments as part of their medical degree. Lesley has concerns about Homer's behaviour around patients, as she feels that he lacks professionalism through his blunt language towards patients, who are visibly distressed. Furthermore, he appears to be quite rough when examining patients on the ward.

How appropriate are each of the following responses by Lesley in this situation?

A. Tell Homer that his behaviour towards patients is not professional and should be improved.

B. Accept that this is Homer's nature with patients and nothing can be done.

C. Alert their supervisor to Homer's lack of professionalism.

D. Suggest to a patient that they tell Homer about his poor bedside manner.

E. Perform some roleplay with Homer, with Lesley as the patient, to allow her to neutrally say that he should be gentler and more professional.

Set 5

Hera is a fourth year medical student shadowing a GP. During a patient consultation, a patient appears to be presenting with some rather peculiar signs and symptoms. Hera recalls reading something online about an illness characterised by these symptoms and thinks she knows what the condition is. The doctor, who doesn't usually engage with medical students during consultations, continues to question the patient regarding their symptoms.

How appropriate are each of the following responses by Hera in this situation?

A. Interrupt the patient's questioning and tell the doctor her diagnosis.

B. Wait until the patient has left the room before telling the doctor her thoughts.

C. Keep her thoughts to herself as the doctor knows best.

D. Signal to the doctor when he finishes his current line of enquiry that she thinks she might know the cause.

E. Write on a post-it note the name of the condition and place it on the desk so the doctor can see it without the patient knowing.

Set 6

Jamie notices Ravi oversees that he is signing another student into a compulsory pathology lecture, so he kindly asks Ravi to keep what he has just witnessed to himself because the other student is busy with a last minute deadline and will attend tomorrow's lecture as it is a repeat of today's but for the biology students. Ravi knows that signing in on behalf of other students is dishonest and that the other student has not alerted the lecturer for permission.

How important to take into account are the following considerations for Ravi when deciding how to respond to the situation?

A. Jamie has kindly asked Ravi to keep what he has just witnessed to himself.

B. He knows the other student has missed many lectures in the past.

C. The other student has not alerted the lecturer for permission

D. The other student plans on attending the same lecture tomorrow.

E. All three students are likely to be disciplined if caught.

Set 7

Dave has been sitting patiently in the surgery's waiting room for an hour to see the doctor. He eventually gets annoyed and starts complaining to Janine, the secretary. Janine asks Dave to calm down and take a seat, at which point he starts shouting at her. Dr Suberwal hears the shouting and walks in.

How important to take into account are the following considerations for Dr Suberwal when deciding how to respond to the situation?

A. Dave is upset

B. Dave is unwell

C. There are a large number of people waiting to be seen

D. Janine feels unsafe

E. Other patients may feel unsafe

Set 8

Myra is a first year medical student who comes to a lecture one day in first term with an eyebrow piercing. She is not aware of the medical school's code of conduct which strongly discourages wearing such items of jewellery. Before the lecture, she bumps into another student who alerts her to the rules of the university. The piercing is new and very expensive, and in order to prevent it from closing up, the stud must stay in.

How important to take into account are the following considerations for Myra when deciding how to respond to the situation?

A. The piercing will close up if she doesn't keep the stud in.

B. The cost of the piercing.

C. That the rule is only in place due to professionalism with regard to patient contact, and first year students only have lectures and tutorials for the first term.

D. That the rule of the medical school must be followed at all times.

E. That the other medical student may be jealous of the eyebrow-piercing.

Set 9

Mark is a final year medical student and notices that a colleague has posted some of their notes into a large, but private group on Facebook to encourage learning amongst other students. In the colleague's notes, she refers to the patient as Mr X although on closer examination of a scanned history, the patient's full name is visible. Mark decides to respond to his colleague's actions.

How important to take into account are the following considerations for Mark when deciding how to respond to the situation?

A. The Facebook post was in a private group

B. The colleague has already been cautioned by the medical school

C. Other colleagues may benefit from the notes and histories

D. The patient's right to confidentiality

E. The colleague was not aware that the patient's name was visible

Set 10

Mandeep and Imran are third year dental students alternating in consultations at one of the dental teaching practices. One patient, who receives a check up with high frequency at the practice, informs Mandeep that in the last session, Imran was bragging about copying an essay from online about hygiene in dentistry for an assignment submitted in their first year. Mandeep knows Imran to be an honest, disciplined and intelligent student, and is aware that this patient has invented rumours about dentists in the past.

How important to take into account are the following considerations for Mandeep when deciding how to respond to the situation?

A. The current reputation of Imran as an honest student in the dental school.

B. The patient's history of inventing rumours about past dentists.

C. The dental school's requirement to report any allegations of plagiarism for essays.

D. That the essay was written in Imran's first year of dental school.

E. The essay title.

Set 11

Edwin, a third year medical student, is entering a lift in the hospital to head to some afternoon bedside teaching. Whilst in the lift, Edwin overhears two junior doctors discussing the results of a CT scan of one of their patients (Mr Ahmed) that showed a strange lump. There are other members of the public inside the lift.

How appropriate are each of the following responses by Edwin in this situation?

1. Speak to the junior doctors once they have left the lift and mention to them that some of the other people in the lift may have heard their discussions about Mr Ahmed's CT scan.

2. Interrupt the junior doctors whilst in the lift and mention to them that they should carry on their conversation in a more private place where only members of the medical team can hear.

3. Ignore the conversation this time and only discuss the issue with the junior doctors if you see them doing the same again.

Set 12

Khadija, a fourth year medical student, is on her GP placement. Today she is sitting in with the Dr Richardson. Dr Richardson is seeing a new patient for the first time and is noting down some important medical information on the computer. Khadija notices that Dr Richardson has mistakenly typed that the patient has no allergies when the patient mentioned an allergy to ibuprofen.

How appropriate are each of the following responses by Khadija in this situation?

1. Ignore the error as Dr Richardson has far more years of clinical experience than Khadija.

2. Politely mention to Dr Richardson once the patient has left the consultation that he may have made a mistake.

3. Report Dr Richardson to the medical school as he is a bad example for students to learn from.

Set 13

Hassan and Steve are two friends in the same year at medical school. Steve is furious about the grades he recently got on a feedback form about his ability to take blood safely and professionally from patients.

How appropriate are each of the following responses by Hassan in this situation?

1. Offer to teach Steve how to take blood safely by practicing on each other at home.
2. Talk to Steve to find out how he feels the procedure went and what he finds unfair about the feedback.
3. Suggest to Steve that he waits a couple of days and then emails his personal tutor to seek advice.
4. Report the consultant to the medical school for unfairly picking on Steve.

Set 14

Matthew and Anna are attending the final lecture of a busy day. Matthew has a football match immediately after the lecture and the lecture is overrunning. Matthew makes a discrete phone call during the lecture to inform his team that he will be late. The professor confronts Matthew and points to a sign showing that mobile phones should not be used inside the lecture theatre. He pauses the lecture and demands Matthew to leave. Meanwhile, other students that were also using their phones in the lecture theatre were allowed to stay.

How important to take into account are the following considerations for Anna when deciding how to respond to the situation?

1. The lecture had overrun 15 minutes longer than scheduled.
2. Matthew tried to be as quiet as possible when making the call, so people were minimally disrupted.
3. The professor made it clear at the start of the academic year that the rules do not tolerate mobile phones during teaching.
4. The other students who used their phones were allowed to remain in the lecture.

Set 15

Three friends, Mary, Sandra and Harry had an argument earlier that day. Sandra reveals to Harry that Mary once copied his essay when she was short of time before a deadline two years ago. Mary is usually very ethical, and this would be out of her normal character. Sandra also has a well-established history at university of creating gossip about fellow students.

How important to take into account are the following considerations for Harry when deciding how to respond to the situation?

A. Mary's reputation amongst her peers if she is caught out having copied Harry's work

B. The essay in question was almost two years ago.

C. Given Sandra's reputation, she may be deliberately lying to cause tension.

D. The medical school issued an email with a zero tolerance to plagiarism at the start of the course

Set 16

Francesca is a medical student with many extracurricular hobbies. She is falling asleep in her outpatient clinic. This is not the first time she has been seen to look very tired and drowsy on placement.

How important to take into account are the following considerations for the supervising doctor when responding to the situation?

A. The patient's perception of the quality of future doctors being trained.

B. Francesca is likely to be missing many learning opportunities that she cannot gather from a textbook.

C. The consultation was a simple follow up appointment, so Francesca did not miss anything special.

D. Francesca has been busy up all the previous night preparing for a presentation she is making at lunch to all the doctors.

Set 17

A patient called Roshan is due for an appendicectomy tomorrow at 9am. Dr Akku was performing routine checks on the patient before the operation tomorrow and realised the team have not checked a vital component of the patient's health which could affect the operation. The lab is currently closed and will open tomorrow at 10am, and therefore bloods can't be analysed before the operation.

Choose both the one most appropriate action and the one least appropriate action that Dr Akku should take in response to this situation.

A. Call the surgical registrar on call as soon as he can

B. Reschedule Roshan's operation for 5pm, but inform him while doing so

C. Reschedule Roshan's operation for the next day, but don't inform him while doing so

Set 18

Michael and John are medical students on their respiratory placement. They've been requested to join the doctors on their ward rounds, however John sees Michael vlogging using his camera for his social media channels, where he daily vlogs. Some patients seem to look frustrated by this.

Choose both the one most appropriate action and the one least appropriate action that John should take in response to this situation.

A. Talk to Michael privately, and remind them of GMC guideline

B. Tell the supervising doctor

C. Give Michael one more week to redeem himself, in the hope they might stop vlogging

Set 19

Alex is the leader of a group project. Chloe comes up to Alex, and complains that Lily isn't contributing to the project, and tends to skip meetings without any explanations. Chloe asks Alex to take action against her.

Choose both the one most appropriate action and the one least appropriate action that Alex should take in response to this situation.

A. Arrange a 1-1 meeting with Lily to explore her reasons to her behaviour

B. Ask Chloe to have a meeting with Lily to sort things out

C. Kick out Lily from the group

Set 20

A 4th year medical student tells the doctor they're attached to that they feel overwhelmed by the amount of work on the ward, and is affecting their mental health.

Choose both the one most appropriate action and the one least appropriate action that the doctor should take in response to this situation.

A. Sit down with the student to explore their concerns, and give them a break

B. Tell them to push a little harder, and that they can leave slightly earlier

C. Tell them to get on with it since NHS is understaffed

Solutions

Q1. A very appropriate thing to do

This immediately allows the patient to justify her statement or appreciate that it has little weighting if she cannot provide concrete explanations of Adele's immaturity. It involves trying to tackle the problem from the roots which is always advised.

Q2. A very appropriate thing to do

Although not an immediate response, this is the most appropriate thing to do when the time is right, to ensure that the nurse, who is a valued member of the medical team, is being listened to.

Q3. A very appropriate thing to do

This is a polite thing to do to alleviate the patient's distress and build a rapport with them as they may have entered with a negative outlook.

Q4. Inappropriate but not awful

Although it doesn't make matters worse, and Adele will understand that the apology is to alleviate the patient's distress, it is still an inappropriate response as the doctor does not give the nurse an opportunity to explain herself.

Q5. Inappropriate but not awful

Although it doesn't make matters worse, and Adele will understand that the apology is to alleviate the patient's distress, it is still an inappropriate response as the doctor does not give the nurse an opportunity to explain herself.

It is important to note that you can have more than one 'very appropriate' or 'inappropriate' response per set.

Set 2

Q1. A very appropriate thing to do

Although he is not the doctor, by allowing Luma to voice her concerns and feel listened to, a level of trust is being established. This rapport could later come in handy if Parth ever feels that something needs to be told to the GP, as Luma would be more easily encouraged to discuss things with the GP, a doctor of greater knowledge.

Q2. A very appropriate thing to do

This would allow the patient to get the best advice regarding her qualms, without Parth needing to breach confidentiality.

Q3. A very inappropriate thing to do

Confidentiality is sometimes referred to as the 5th key principle of ethics in medicine (after Autonomy, Beneficence, Non-maleficence and Justice). Parth would be breaking patient confidentiality if this were the case, as Luma would have told Dr Morris herself had she wanted to. Without Luma's consent, Parth would be making matters worse, although Dr Morris would of course still keep the information confidential.

Q4. A very inappropriate thing to do

A key quality regarding the good medical practice of doctors, described by the GMC, is probity. This response lacks probity as it is a dishonest deed. Parth may be incorrect in his assumptions, and an error in communication may have resulted in Luma receiving the wrong prescription. As a result, it would be Parth's duty to follow this up with the patient and ensure everything was correct.

Q5. A very inappropriate thing to do

Confidentiality is sometimes referred to as the 5th key principle of ethics in medicine (after Autonomy, Beneficence, Non-maleficence and Justice). Parth would be violating the patient's privacy by looking at her records without consent, due to his position as a medical student, as opposed to a clinical professional involved in her care.

Set 3

Q1. A very inappropriate thing to do

Local resolution is always preferred when it is possible. There is clearly a problem that can be resolved in this situation and reporting the doctor to the GMC will not help alleviate it. Verily, it may make matters worse, blowing things out of proportion and affecting Dr. George when he is at his most vulnerable.

Q2. A very inappropriate thing to do

This involves detaching himself from the situation, which would often not be an awful thing, just inappropriate. However, the secretary has told Dr. Fred this especially as patients' lives are being put in danger, and by not doing anything in this instance, the problem will continue to be exacerbated. Melissa clearly feels as though another doctor must speak to him.

Q3. A very appropriate thing to do

This involves tackling the problem at its roots and dealing with it instantaneously. Offering time off can also be helpful to improve Dr. George's attitude and help him overcome the grief.

Q4. A very inappropriate thing to do

This is dishonesty as Dr. George hasn't investigated the situation further, despite patient complaints. This only serves to make matters worse as Dr. George may continue to make mistakes and potentially keep drinking.

Q5. A very appropriate thing to do

This would strongly be advised to ensure that the patients' complaints are valid and may help corroborate Melissa's concerns. From here, Dr. Fred will be able to take the next steps to alleviating the problem.

Q1. A very appropriate thing to do

As brutally honest as this sounds, it may sound offensive perhaps, but Homer would be expected to take on the constructive criticism acknowledging that Lesley is doing it for his improvement in clinical care provision.

Q2. A very inappropriate thing to do

Usually, this would be considered inappropriate but not awful because the response is merely a lack of action. However, when this lack of action makes matters worse, i.e. patients being visibly distressed around this student, then it is considered very inappropriate.

Q3. Inappropriate but not awful

This would not be a good response as local resolution is preferred for minor conflict. Ultimately, however, Homer would be told about the improvements that he must make in his behaviour, so the result isn't awful.

Q4. A very inappropriate thing to do

This would not be recommended as it would undermine Homer's ability and reduce the patient's faith in medical students and quite possibly even the profession.

Q5. A very appropriate thing to do

In doing this, Homer will find Lesley's advice and criticism more believable and constructive. This, like advising another person about their behaviour in the presence of the one who is in the wrong, is a polite way of teaching good manners in the medical profession.

Set 5

Q1. A very inappropriate thing to do

Not only is this poor etiquette that disrupts the patient-doctor relationship, it also undermines the knowledge of the doctor and reduces the trust the patient will have in the doctor, ultimately making matters worse. It lacks subtlety and tact and could be carried out in a much more delicate way.

Q2. A very inappropriate thing to do

Although this response may be subtle and professional as Hera is not openly undermining the doctor's intelligence, the fact that it is so slow that the patient has left the room without being correctly diagnosed may be putting their life in danger. Thus, it is a very inappropriate response.

Q3. A very inappropriate thing to do

This may make matters worse, as the patient's life may be put in jeopardy, especially if the condition has immediate short-term effects that may need to be tended to. It may simply be that this condition slipped the doctor's mind. She should mention what she thinks may be going on but at a suitable time.

Q4. A very appropriate thing to do

This is a relatively subtle thing to do and maintains professionalism. In addition, it allows the doctor to be made aware of Hera's thoughts without blatantly interrupting the consultation, maintaining the doctor-patient engagement.

Q5. A very appropriate thing to do

This is a very subtle thing to do and maintains professionalism. In addition, it allows the doctor to be made aware of Hera's thoughts without interrupting the consultation, maintaining the doctor-patient engagement.

Set 6

Q1. Not important at all

Having witnessed a dishonest action, however kindly Jamie has asked, Ravi must inform the lecturer of what has taken place.

Q2. Not important at all

This is not relevant to the problem that has taken place. Ravi should not take the role of the medical school as judging whether the other student is fit to practise medicine.

Q3. Very important

This is a severe lack of professionalism from the student and must be taken into account giving reason for Ravi to report the situation.

Q4. Of minor importance

It is possible that this alleviates the matter pertaining to Jamie's wrongdoing, but it would still be required that Ravi alert the lecturer of what has taken place.

Q5. Very important

The students should be wary of the consequences of such actions, and this should prevent them from committing them. Medical schools issue strict guidelines about the incorrect nature of such fraudulent activity.

Set 7

Q1. Important

It is definitely important to acknowledge that Dave is upset in this situation, however this is not vital to dealing with the situation, because it doesn't excuse his verbally abusive behaviour. If Dr Suberwal were to focus on dealing with Dave's feelings, she would not be dealing with the situation properly and preventing such intolerable behaviour.

Q2. Important

It is definitely important to acknowledge that Dave is not feeling well, hence why he is in the surgery, however this is not vital as it doesn't excuse his verbally abusive behaviour. If Dr Suberwal were to focus on dealing with Dave's illness at the time of the shouting, she would not be dealing with the situation properly and preventing such intolerable behaviour.

Q3. Of minor importance

This doesn't have a huge impact in terms of dealing with the patient shouting at Janine. If anything, it could be considered by Dr Suberwal, who may wish to call the patient in immediately in order to calm him down.

Q4. Very important

This is the major issue that is of primary concern at the moment and is the reason as to why the doctor must respond to the situation. If the secretary's safety wasn't at risk, then it would not be as big an issue.

Q5. Very important

This is a major issue of primary concern at the moment and is one of the main reasons as to why the doctor must respond to the situation. If other patients don't feel safe, then it must be resolved immediately and so this should definitely be taken into account.

Set 8

Q1. Not important at all

This should not be considered when the rules clearly state that eyebrow-piercings are not permitted in the medical school. Therefore, the piercing will have to close as she will not be allowed to wear an eyebrow-piercing anyway.

Q2. Not important at all

Myra must take responsibility for the fact that she is not adhering to the rules stipulated in the medical school's code of conduct, and unfortunately remove the piercing and accept this loss of money.

Q3. Very important

The context of the rule is very important to consider: If this is true about the patient contact, then it allows Myra to keep the piercing in.

Q4. Very important

If this is indeed the case, then Myra must stick to the medical school's code of conduct and take out the piercing.

Q5. Not important at all

This may or may not be true, but regardless should not affect Myra's decision to adhere to the medical school's rules.

Q1. Not important at all

By posting the patient's details to be viewed by other medical students, patient confidentiality has been breached, which is key to this issue.

Q2. Of minor importance

This should not affect Mark's decision to respond appropriately, because if anything, the colleague is risky in their actions. It would be up to the medical board or the university to decide whether the prior incidence was relevant to this one.

Q3. Of minor importance

Although the colleague may have had pure intentions, the patient's confidentiality has still been breached. However, this may be taken into account by Mark when reporting the incidence.

Q4. Very important

Confidential medical care is central to doctor-patient trust and recognised in law as being in the public interest. The fact that people are encouraged to seek advice and treatment, including for communicable diseases, benefits society as a whole as well as the individual.

Q5. Of minor importance

Whether the colleague intended to post patient-identifiable data or not is irrelevant and not at all important. This situation is about whether or not Mark raises what he has noticed and ensures that it is taken down.

Set 10

Q1. Not important at all

This is not down to Mandeep to take into consideration, it is for the dental school. The question at hand is whether Mandeep should take this into account when deciding whether or not to inform the dental school about Imran's potential wrongdoing.

Q2. Of minor importance

Although, Mandeep should not try to be the detective in this situation, it is important that he establishes whether or not the patient is telling the truth with regard to this allegation, before potentially tarnishing Imran's reputation, and escalating the matter by taking it to the dental school.

Q3. Very important

If the dental school has issued guideline or a code of conduct about something, it is always very important to adhere to.

Q4. Not important at all

Whether the essay was submitted in first year of the dental school or in the current year of study, if it were indeed the case and the dental school has guidelines pertaining to the matter, then this definitely should not be taken into consideration, as appropriate action must be carried, and justice served.

Q5. Not important at all

Whatever the topic of the essay, plagiarism is a serious allegation due to the dishonesty of the student, so this should definitely not be taken into account. Rather, Mandeep must respond to the issue of cheating itself.

Set 11

Q1. The correct answer is very appropriate. This is a sensible action for the medical student to take and addresses at least one aspect of the situation. It is important to remind professionals to maintain patient confidentiality at all times.

Q2. The correct answer is very appropriate. This action again is reasonable to take. Not only does it address the situation but by mentioning this whilst inside the lift may restore confidence in the overhearing members of the public.

Q3. The correct answer is inappropriate, but not awful. The error made by the junior doctors should not go unnoticed. This type of error should not be allowed to reoccur, as the potential repercussions of breaking confidentiality are considerable. Ignoring the situation altogether does not make this specific incident worse; hence the answer is not very inappropriate.

Set 12

Q1. The correct answer is a very inappropriate thing to do. By ignoring a potentially fatal error Khadija is likely to be making the situation worse.

Q2. The correct answer is very appropriate thing to do. This addresses the situation and helps the doctor understand that they may have made a mistake. By being polite and telling the doctor as soon as the consultation is over Khadija is acting professionally and also helping avoid a potentially fatal error whilst not reducing the trust the patient may have in the doctor.

Q3. The correct answer is a very inappropriate thing to do. Whilst the mistake made by the doctor is potentially dangerous, it is unjustifiable to go immediately to the medical school to report this issue. It is best to deal with issues at a local level as oppose to reporting them straight away to the medical school which may make the situation worse.

Set 13

Q1. The correct answer is a very inappropriate thing to do. Although Hassan is trying to help Steve improve his blood taking ability, it is unprofessional to be practicing on each other without supervision, especially outside of a clinical environment. There is also a big risk of how they dispose of any needles. Therefore, this will make the situation worse, so the answer is inappropriate.

Q2. The correct answer is a very appropriate thing to do. This is a very reasonable thing for Hassan to do to try and gather more information from Steve. It is subtle, timely and professional. Perhaps he may be able to also share some personal tips and reassurance to Steve to help address the situation.

Q3. The correct answer is appropriate, but not ideal. Whilst it is a good thing to inform your personal tutor when you receive any feedback (both positive or negative), this should occur as soon as possible particularly in the case of receiving negative feedback which could benefit from extra supervision to avoid putting patients at risk.

Q4. The correct answer is a very inappropriate thing to do. The consultant has a role in providing feedback to medical students to help improve their clinical practice. Even if Steve feels hard done by it would be inappropriate to report the consultant to the medical school straight away. Issues are best resolved at a local level first before escalating them.

Set 14

1. This is not important at all. This is because regardless of whether the lecture is running on time or is running late the rules of the medical school still need to be respected. Therefore, we should not take this piece of information into account.

2. This is of minor importance. The university code of conduct is clear that mobile phones are not to be used in the lecture theatre. It therefore does not matter to us how loud the conversation is. This information is something that could be taken into account, but it does not matter if it is considered or not.

3. This is very important. Medical students must always follow any rules and guidelines that are set out by their university. Therefore, it is vital that we consider this information.

4. This is important. It is important that all students are treated evenly so we should take this information into account. However, it still does not justify Matthew's use of his phone and it is not vital for Anna to take this information into account (as per the official definitions)

Set 15

1. This is not important at all. Plagiarism is not tolerable in any situation. If we worry about Mary's reputation suffering as a consequence of this wrongdoing, we will be neglecting a serious offence. This information should not be taken into account at all.

2. This is not important at all. Plagiarism is not tolerable in any situation. The time frame is also irrelevant as the issue should be addressed even if the incident was occurred many years ago to prevent it from reoccurring in the future.

3. This is important. It is important that we don't falsely accuse Mary of a serious incident especially given that this accusation occurred following a recent argument. However, equally we cannot just assume that this is a false rumour, especially when the accusation is so severe.

4. This is very important. It is vital to take this information into account because any breaking of rules issued by the medical school would constitute a serious offence.

1. This is very important. It is vital to protect the reputation of the medical profession in the public eye. It is completely unacceptable to fall asleep in a patient consultation and shows a lack of professionalism.

2. This is very important. Medical students are privileged to be able to observe patient consultations. A textbook cannot demonstrate many of the things that can be learnt in person from observing the doctor-patient conversation and physical examination. Missing out on this learning may potentially endanger future patients assessed by the medical student.

3. This is not important at all. We should not try to use this information to justify a tired medical student falling asleep. It is unprofessional behaviour regardless of how educational the consultation is.

4. This is of minor importance. Having this information does not alter how we respond to her unprofessional behaviour. Perhaps, she may be providing a learning opportunity to many doctors at lunch, but this does not justify falling asleep. Therefore, this information is something that could be taken into account, but it does not matter if it is considered or not.

Set 17

Calling the surgical registrar **(A)** is the most appropriate action; it will allow Dr Akku to check if the test was missed due by accident or on purpose. It also escalates the issue and allows an experienced doctor to provide guidance on how to proceed rather than erroneously making a rash decision like rescheduling the operation. Even worse is rescheduling the operation AND not notifying the patient **(C)** as that goes completely against the principles of transparency and will also cause logistical issues if the patient turns up (or doesn't!) on the wrong day.

Set 18

Speak to Michael and reminding him about GMC guidelines **(A)** is the most appropriate action - it allows Michael to be educated about GMC guidelines and gives him a clear opportunity to change his behaviour. Informing the supervising doctor **(B)** is not terrible but also not the best course of action as ultimately, this issue should only be escalated if Michael continues to breach patient confidentiality and make patients uncomfortable. It is not appropriate to escalate the issue **(B)** without at least giving Michael the chance to change. Simply waiting for change to happen with no intervention **(C)** is the least appropriate course of action as it's unlikely that Michael would stop vlogging and it ignores the issues surrounding patient comfort and confidentiality.

Set 19

In general, in the SJT, it is good practice to explore and ask questions rather than rushing into things. This is a great example questions that demonstrates this. Exploring Chloe's concerns **(A)** is the most appropriate approach given that it will allow Alex to assimilate more information before making a decision (it is not wise to make decisions after only hearing one side of the story after all!). Whilst asking Chloe and Lily to resolve the situation between themselves **(B)** is understandable, it ignores the fact that Alex is the group leader and hence, has a responsibility to at least understand Chloe's concerns. Kicking Lily from the group **(C)** is the least appropriate given that Alex has not heard her side of the story and is making a judgement on limited information.

Set 20

Similarly to Set 19, this question is all about exploring so unsurprisingly; option **(A)** is the most appropriate as it allows the doctor to understand what the student is finding difficult and take steps to try to help. Telling them to 'push harder' **(B)** is a response that demonstrates a lack of empathy and is premature without knowing the facts of the matter. Finally, telling them to 'get on with it' **(C)** is even worse as it completely ignores the student's cry for health and dismisses their mental health concerns.

What next?

When should I book the test?

• Give yourself 3-4 weeks to prepare. Unless you have other plans during summer, a month (assuming you finish school on the 21st July) is a good amount of time to prepare. It doesn't matter when you book the test, but during September, you'll have school again. Whenever you book it, allow yourself 3-4 weeks to prepare at the very least.

• Book the test at the time of day you're most effective. If you're a morning person and you know you perform better in the early hours - book the test then. At the same time, it's good to give yourself a few hours before the exam to clear your mind and run through the key strategies. This isn't a content-based exam, so don't bother cramming anything. Instead, you should remind yourself of the different steps and techniques used to approach each subtest.

What should I do on the day of the exam?

• Run through the 'basics'. By the time you take the exam, you'll hopefully have had enough practice, and in the morning (or the day before), try to run through the key strategies and approaches for each subtest. Remind yourself to remove any bad habits such as over-thinking and automatically reaching for the calculator for the simple sums.

• Limit how much you drink 2 hours before the exam. The exam won't be paused if you require a toilet break. Don't take the risk - keep hydrated but don't drink too much.

• Arrive at least 15 minutes before your scheduled test time. You'll need to 'check-in' before you take the test, and it's always a good idea to allow yourself some extra time in case any problems arise.

• Ensure you're comfortable with the instructions and protocol. It's best to know exactly what's going to happen on the day, both before and during the exam - you want to minimise any distractions and remove unexpected surprises. All the information can be found on the UCAT website: http://www.ucat.ac.uk/test-day

• Have a screenshot or printed copy of the email confirmation handy as well

• Make sure you double check the route and try to visit the centre at least once before!

• Be confident. You're already more prepared than the students who haven't been on a course such as this one - the strategies and approaches we teach you are designed to save you time and boost your score. If you've practised hard and integrated many of the strategies in our course, you'll have a good chance of getting a strong score. Even if you're preparing a bit late, there is loads of useful information in this course that you can apply straight away.

• Get into the 'zone' and enjoy the process. It's normal to feel scared, stressed, and highly anxious before a big exam like the UCAT. We shouldn't take away from the importance of the UCAT, but at the end of the day, the UCAT isn't essential for a successful application - you can choose where you apply after you get your score. Don't focus on the outcome: view the UCAT as an exciting step towards the next stage in your life, whether you do well or not. You can deal with the repercussions of a poor score if you really do end up doing badly, but on test-day, you should be focused, have a clear mind, and aim to put everything you've worked on into practice.

Anything I should know about the test centre?

- Reduce distractions by putting on earplugs/headphones. You'll be given earplugs or headphones when entering the test room. Consider putting these on, especially if you think you'll be distracted by other test-takers.
- Check the permanent markers work before starting the test. Everyone makes mistakes, so ensure the markers are working.
- Ask for more than one whiteboard if they let you. Try asking for more than one whiteboard before you start - unless you have really small writing, you'll probably run out of space. Not all centres will hand them out, but it's worth a try.

What to bring on the day?

- Identification. Ensure you have the right ID, otherwise you'll be turned away and lose your test fee. Valid forms of ID include a current passport and a current driving license.
- Bring some water, but no food or drink inside in the test room. It's a long exam (2 hours), and you'll probably want to be refreshed and hydrated before you walk in.
- Always check the instructions on the email confirmation in case they add anything else to bring.

The 6med Promise

If you require help, please contact us - we're not here just to teach you the UCAT.

Below are some of the common things students always ask us about, and we urge you to do so if you want any help. What happens if:

- **You get a good score**. This is hopefully the case for most of you, but you still need to be careful which universities you apply to. Some universities don't place much emphasis on the UCAT, so if the rest of your application is standard, or below average, you may not want to apply to such places.

- **You get a weak score**. This can happen to anyone, and whatever the reason, there's no point worrying about it. You must submit an application built around your strongest areas, so ensure you choose the four medical schools which best suit your strengths, as well as your personal preferences.

- **You're struggling to write a good personal statement**. Some students underestimate how crucial the personal statement can be. The personal statement is your 'front door' - it advertises who you are and the qualities you claim to possess. We know students who have been selected for interview before BMAT results day because their personal statements were so powerful. We got so many question about this we've actually launched a brand new personal statement course and book really recently, as well as upgrading our editing service- so do take a look on the website if you're stuck!

- **You have an interview**. If the personal statement is your 'front door', then the interview is the person (you) who opens the door. It's hard to hide during an interview, and they can be very difficult. At the same time, no matter how scary an interview can be, interviewers are still just examining and marking candidates from a checklist with set criteria - you must understand what they're looking for, and how best to get the right boxes ticked. Your tutors obviously can't provide one-on-one tuition for all of you, but they'll be happy to give you as much advice as they can. The things that can potentially come up are skills and values you'll further develop at medical school: ethical awareness, professional conduct, communication skills, etc. Our tutors will be well acquainted with the areas you should be working on.

- **You have an offer**. The road to medical school is near completion, and for the luckier among you, it may be hard deciding between different universities. This is mostly a personal decision, but you may want a realistic representation of the teaching and opportunities at these medical schools. Ask your tutors for more information about their medical school - they may even have a few friends in other medical schools who could help.

- If you'd like to get in touch, please visit the Contact page on the 6med website - we'd love to hear from you!

Closing Remarks

Congratulations on reaching the end of this course! We're delighted that you took this part of the journey with us, and sincerely hope that we've been of some help.

Unfortunately, there's still a long way to go before you can relax. The UCAT is a demanding exam that plays a potentially huge part in your medical school application, so don't get complacent. Keep on doing those practice questions, keep on honing your skills, and take the exam with confidence - no matter how well you do, you know that you've done your best, and that's all anyone can ask for.

Remember, if there's absolutely anything you need at all, please don't hesitate to get in touch. We were in the same position as you a few years ago, and the help we got from older students was instrumental in helping us get into medical school - we would be more than happy to return the favour. If you need help with personal statements, interviews, or anything else really, just shoot your tutors an email (they should give it to you in the course), and they'll be happy to help.

If you think our course helped, and you're taking BMAT, come along to one our BMAT courses in September and October (www.bmatcrashcourse.com)!
Also, if (and when) you get called up for interviews, you might be interested in our Interview Crash Course (www.interviewcrashcourse.com).
If you're still writing your personal statement - we've got a course and a book for that too!

All that's really left is to wish you the very best of luck with the UCAT and your application!

UCAT · NINJA

UCAT.NINJA MAKES PREPARING FOR THE UCAT AS PAINLESS AS IT CAN BE.

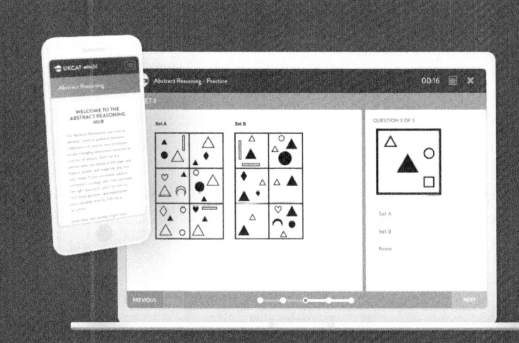

WHY UCAT NINJA

Start With The Technique. For each section of the UCAT, we have strategy and technique tutorials to get you prepared for practice questions.

Access To 2,000+ Practice Questions. UCAT.Ninja gives you access to hundreds questions for each section, along with fully worked solutions.

Realistic Exam Runs. We've devised full mock exams, delivered in the on-screen format as the real exam for an accurate exam experience.

Designed and delivered by Oxbridge medics.

———

Your expert online preparation tool.

Improve your score rapidly

Unlimited access on any plan

We offer bursaries

Fantastic. I used your UCAT.Ninja service and scored a 747 (Band 1 SJT) and couldn't have done it without you guys!

Lucy

www.UKCAT.NINJA

Printed in Great Britain
by Amazon

82307085R00174